Lessons Learned at 40

A Journey of Growth and Self-Discovery

by

Yolanda Trevino

First Edition

Lightbody Publishing

P.O. Box 151 Lafayette, CA, USA

Copyright © 2023 by Yolanda Trevino. All rights reserved.

Published by Lightbody Publishing, LLC

P.O. Box 151

Lafayette, CA 94549

www.lightbodypublishing.com

First Edition: August 8, 2023

ISBN: 978-1-7371595-4-4

This book is a personal account of the author's experiences and reflections on personal growth and development. The views and opinions expressed in this book are those of the author and do not necessarily reflect the official policy or position of any organization or institution. The author has made every effort to ensure the accuracy and completeness of the information presented in this book, but makes no warranties or representations as to the accuracy or completeness of the information provided. The reader is solely responsible for any actions or decisions taken based on the information contained in this book.

The information contained in this book is for educational and informational purposes only and is not intended as medical advice. The information in this book should not be used to diagnose, treat, or prevent any disease or health condition. Always consult with a qualified healthcare professional before starting any diet, exercise, or supplement program, or before taking any medication.

The author and publisher specifically disclaim all responsibility for any liability, loss, or risk, personal or otherwise, which is incurred as a consequence, directly or indirectly, of the use and application of any of the contents of this book. This book is designed to provide general information on personal growth and development and is not intended to serve as medical, legal, or financial advice. The author and publisher are not responsible for any actions taken by readers based on the information provided in this book.

Readers are encouraged to seek out the advice of qualified professionals in the relevant fields for personalized guidance. The exercises and practices presented in this book are intended to support personal growth and well-being, but individual results may vary. The author and publisher do not guarantee any specific outcomes or results from the use of the information provided in this book.

All rights are reserved. No part of this book may be reproduced, stored in a retrieval system, or transmitted in any form or by any means, electronic, mechanical, photocopying, recording, or otherwise, without the prior written permission of the author and the publisher. Any unauthorized use, sharing, reproduction, or distribution of this book or its contents is strictly prohibited and may result in legal action.

Lessons Learned at 40: A Journey of Growth and Self-Discovery and Lightbody Publishing LLC, are trademarks of Yolanda Trevino. All other trademarks are the property of their respective owners.

Dedication

To all those who have helped me become the person I am today, and to those who are still searching for their own path. May this book offer you the insights and perspective you need to overcome obstacles and find your way.

Table of Contents

Preface 1

Introduction 3

1. The Power of Self-Care: What I Wish I Knew by 40 5
2. Prioritizing Health, Wellness and Relationships for Long-Term Success: What I Wish I Knew By 40 12
3. Building and Maintaining Healthy Relationships: What I Wish I Knew by 40 16
4. Balancing Work and Personal Life for Greater Fulfillment: What I Wish I Knew by 40 21
5. Coping with Loss and Overcoming Adversity: What I Wish I Knew by 40 27
6. Embracing Your Authentic Self and Finding Your Voice: What I Wish I Knew By 40 34
7. Tips for Managing Finances and Planning for the Future: What I Wish I Knew by 40 42
8. Finding Joy and Meaning in Everyday Life: What I Wish I Knew by 40 48
9. Navigating Career Changes and Finding Your Purpose: What I Wish I Knew by 40 53
10. Letting Go of Perfectionism: What I Wish I Knew by 40 63
11. Overcoming Fear: What I Wish I Knew by 40 70
12. The Importance of Communication: What I Wish I Knew by 40 75
13. Setting Realistic Expectations: What I Wish I Knew by 40 80
14. Self-Advocacy: What I Wish I Knew by 40 84
15. Cultivating Resilience: What I Wish I Knew by 40 89
16. Building a Support System: What I Wish I Knew by 40 94

17. The Power of Gratitude: What I Wish I Knew by 40 100

18. Developing a Growth Mindset: What I Wish I Knew by 40 105

19. Finding Your Purpose: What I Wish I Knew by 40 112

20. Finding Joy in the Journey: What I Wish I Knew by 40 118

21. Learning to Let Go: What I Wish I Knew by 40 123

22. Creating Healthy Habits: What I Wish I Knew by 40 130

Reflection Questions for Personal Growth and Self-Discovery 135

7 Exercises for Cultivating Mindfulness, Self-Awareness, and Growth . 139

Conclusion 142

Acknowledgements 144

Preface

Welcome to Lessons Learned at 40: A Journey of Growth and Self-Discovery. This book is a reflection of my personal experiences and lessons learned over the years, with the hope of inspiring and encouraging readers to reflect on their own journey of personal growth and self-discovery.

At 40, I reached a turning point in my life that inspired me to take a deeper look at who I was and who I wanted to be. I began to think about all the things I wished I had known when I was younger, and how those lessons could have helped me avoid some of the challenges and struggles I faced in life. With this in mind, I set out to document my journey and share my insights with others who may be on a similar path.

In these pages, you'll find a collection of essays that explore a variety of topics related to personal growth and self-improvement. Each essay includes my personal reflections on the topic, as well as practical advice and tips for putting those lessons into practice.

I've also included reflection questions at the end of each essay to help you delve deeper into the topics and explore how they relate to your own life. Additionally, there's a list of reflection questions and exercises at the end of the book for you to try that can help cultivate mindfulness, self-awareness, and a growth mindset.

I hope that Lessons Learned at 40 will provide you with the insights, inspiration, and tools you need to embark on your own journey of growth and self-discovery. Remember, the journey is just as important as the destination, and every step you take brings you closer to becoming the best version of yourself.

Thank you for taking the time to read this book, and I wish you all the best on your journey.

Warmly,

Yolanda Trevino

Introduction

Welcome to Lessons Learned at 40: A Journey of Growth and Self-Discovery. This book is a collection of essays written from my personal perspective on lessons I wish I knew by 40. I share personal anecdotes and experiences, highlighting the challenges I've faced and the lessons and experiences I've learned throughout my life. From the importance of self-care to finding your purpose in life, each essay covers a different aspect of personal growth and offers practical advice to help you achieve your goals.

As the founder of Evolutionary Body System, a program designed to help people transform their lives through healthy habits and self-discovery, I'm excited to share my journey with you and offer insights and tips to help you navigate your own. From overcoming fear and building resilience to cultivating healthy habits and finding your purpose, these essays cover a wide range of topics that women of all ages can relate to. Whether you're in your 20s, 30s, or 40s, these insights can help you navigate the challenges that come with each stage of life.

As you read through these essays, I invite you to reflect on your own experiences and have included reflection questions at the end of each essay that are designed to help you apply the insights shared to your own life. Whether you're looking to build healthier relationships, find greater fulfillment in your career, or cultivate a more positive mindset, these essays offer guidance and inspiration to help you on your journey.

You'll also find a list of exercises at the conclusion to help you cultivate mindfulness, self-awareness, and a growth mindset. These exercises are designed to support you in your personal growth journey and can be completed at your own pace and in your own time.

It is my hope that this book will inspire and empower you to embrace your journey, learn from your experiences, and discover the beauty in the lessons learned. So, sit back, grab a cup of tea, and join me on this journey of growth and self-discovery.

The Power of Self-Care: What I Wish I Knew by 40

In the first essay of this book, I want to share a personal story about the significance of self-care and self-love and how prioritizing my own well-being has transformed my life. As I reflect on my journey, there's one crucial lesson I wish I had known earlier: the profound importance of both self-care and self-love.

For a long time, I placed other people and matters above myself, neglecting my physical, mental, and emotional well-being. It wasn't until I hit rock bottom that I realized the essentiality of prioritizing myself. Through my path of healing and self-discovery, I learned the power of self-care and how it can catalyze a transformative change. Let me share with you how incorporating these elements can profoundly benefit your own life.

As a young adult, I grappled with low self-esteem and a negative body image, leading to battles with unhealthy behaviors well into adulthood. Externally, I projected an air of confidence, concealing my internal struggles. However, I lacked self-compassion and sought refuge in destructive habits to cope or maintain control in my life. The turning point came when I hit rock bottom and sought help, discovering the profound impact of self-care and self-love. Through practicing meditation and seeking talk therapy, I began understanding the significance of prioritizing my physical and mental health. Taking small steps, like exercising regularly and speaking kindly to myself, enabled me to rebuild my confidence and learn to cherish myself for who I am. Though it took time to establish lasting changes, investing in my overall well-being has profoundly transformed my life, and I have emerged as a happier, healthier version of myself.

Self-care is a term often used, but what does it genuinely entail? To me, self-care is an act of self-love, intentionally tending to one's physical, mental, and emotional well-being. It's about being proactive, ensuring you are at your best, rather than just responding to problems as they arise.

Having struggled with weight, trauma, and emotional well-being, I comprehend the ease of neglecting self-care amidst difficult issues. When facing challenges, it becomes effortless to prioritize other matters above ourselves. Yet, the truth is, taking care of ourselves is not only important but also vital for a fulfilling life.

Initially, I wish I had known that self-care goes beyond indulging in bubble baths and massages. While those can be part of it, genuine self-care involves holistic well-being. It includes getting enough sleep, nourishing your body with nutritious food, exercising, and addressing your mental and emotional health.

For me, prioritizing my physical health marked the first step toward a happier life. As I made exercise and proper nutrition a priority, I experienced a sense of well-being I hadn't felt in years. It required consistent effort, but over time, I was able to transform both my body and my life.

Furthermore, I learned that mental and emotional health are equally vital aspects of self-care. Seeking therapy was instrumental in my journey. Addressing my anxiety and depression became more manageable through the guidance of a therapist and I gained a repertoire of practices to manage distress, fostering a sense of tranquility and inner peace.

Another revelation on my path was the power of mindfulness which I learned by practicing mindfulness meditation. Being present and aware of my thoughts and feelings, without judgment, brought significant stress and anxiety relief. Embracing mindfulness practices has greatly improved my mental health and enriched my relationships and life experiences.

It's essential to acknowledge that self-care is not a one-size-fits-all approach. Each person's journey is unique, and what works for one might not work for another. The key is to discover what genuinely resonates with you and prioritize it in your life. For me, it means cherishing my workouts, consuming nourishing food, practicing mindfulness, and setting aside "me time." For someone else, it might entail entirely different aspects.

Lastly, I wish I had realized that self-care is an investment in our future selves. By taking care of ourselves now, we pave the way for a healthier and happier future and enriched life. This becomes even more critical as we age, as investing in our physical, mental, and emotional health can help us to prevent chronic illnesses and mental health issues down the road.

Self-love, on the other hand, involves nurturing a positive and compassionate relationship with ourselves. It entails treating ourselves with kindness, respect, and empathy, recognizing our intrinsic worth and not seeking validation solely from external sources. As we cultivate self-love and compassion, we develop a deeper understanding of ourselves, which also enhances our ability to empathize and understand others.

Among the myriad benefits of self-care and self-love is their ability to help us manage stress and anxiety effectively. Prioritizing ourselves reduces susceptibility to burnout and stress-related health problems. By showing love and compassion to ourselves, we become better equipped to handle life's challenges.

Moreover, practicing self-care and self-love empowers us to establish healthy boundaries and cultivate self-respect. By putting ourselves first, we develop self-esteem and self-confidence, essential components of a fulfilling and meaningful life.

Incorporating self-care and self-love into our daily routines is pivotal. Here are a few simple tips to get started:

1. Prioritize sleep: Ensure you get 7-8 hours of restful sleep each night and create a relaxing bedtime routine.

2. Practice mindfulness: Engage in activities that help you be present in the moment, such as meditation, deep breathing, or yoga.

3. Schedule "me time": Set aside time for activities you enjoy, like reading, painting, or taking a nature walk.

4. Nourish your body: Consume a balanced, nutrient rich diet and stay hydrated to improve your emotional and physical health.

5. Surround yourself with positivity: Spend time with uplifting and supportive people, and engage in activities that bring you joy.

In conclusion, self-care and self-love are indispensable aspects of a fulfilling life. They extend beyond mere indulgences and represent a holistic commitment to our well-being. By prioritizing self-care, we invest in our future and create a pathway to a healthier, happier life. If I had understood this earlier, perhaps some of the struggles I faced could have been avoided. Nevertheless, I am grateful for the lesson learned, and moving forward, I will continue to make self-care a priority.

As you read through this essay, take a moment to reflect on your current self-care and self-love practices. Consider how you can incorporate more of these practices into your daily routine to enhance your overall well-being. Remember, there is no one-size-fits-all approach; find what works for you and nurture your relationship with yourself. By doing so, you will be making a significant investment in your future and paving the way to a healthier, happier life.

Transition

As we discovered in the previous essay, prioritizing self-care and self-love is a fundamental aspect of leading a fulfilling life. However, it's equally vital to recognize that our physical health is as significant as our mental and emotional well-being. Building upon this understanding, the subsequent essay delves into the significance of prioritizing our overall health and wellness, alongside cultivating healthy relationships, as integral contributors to our overall well-being and long-term success. Throughout this essay, we'll explore practical tips for nurturing both our physical and emotional selves, as well as for fostering and sustaining positive relationships. By investing in our health and relationships, we are paving the way for a happier, more rewarding future. So, let's embark on this journey to explore the realms of health, wellness, and relationships, and learn how to make them central priorities in our lives.

Prioritizing Health, Wellness and Relationships for Long-Term Success: What I Wish I Knew By 40

As we journey through life, it becomes increasingly crucial to prioritize our physical and mental well-being. Neglecting our health can lead to various health issues, which can impede our ability to achieve long-term success in all aspects of our lives. This is a lesson I personally learned when I reached my 40s.

For many years, I had placed my well-being on the back burner, focusing instead on unfulfilling relationships, work and various other responsibilities neglecting my own well-being in the process. However, as I started facing health problems, I realized the need for necessary change. I began prioritizing my well-being by incorporating regular exercise, nourishing my body with healthy food, managing stress effectively, and ensuring routine check-ups with my healthcare provider. Through these positive changes, I not only experienced improvements in my physical health but also recognized the importance of cultivating healthy relationships with the people in my life. As a result, I made the courageous decision to distance myself from individuals who not only caused me stress and mental health issues but also contributed to physical problems. Instead, I focused on nurturing relationships that were supportive and uplifting, creating a more conducive environment for personal growth and self-discovery. This shift has significantly improved my overall well-being and happiness.

Healthy relationships are built upon the pillars of respect, communication, and empathy. By taking care of ourselves, we create a positive ripple effect in our interactions with others. When we make time for self-care, we enhance our ability to express our needs and emotions to others while setting healthy boundaries that safeguard our well-being.

Here are some practical steps you can take to prioritize your physical and mental well-being:

1. Make time for exercise: Regular physical activity is vital for maintaining good health. Even dedicating just 30 minutes a day to moderate activity, such as walking, can make a significant difference. Schedule it into your calendar and treat it as you would any other essential appointment.

2. Eat a balanced diet: I can not stress this enough. The food we consume fuels our body and our mind, so making healthy choices is crucial. Aim for a balanced diet filled with nutrients

that includes plenty of fruits, vegetables, lean protein, and whole grains. If you can eat organically, that is best. Stay hydrated by drinking ample water throughout the day.

3. Get enough sleep: Adequate sleep is essential for our physical and mental well-being. Strive for seven to eight hours of sleep each night and create a relaxing bedtime routine to wind down effectively.

4. Practice stress-reduction techniques: Chronic stress can adversely affect our overall health, so it's essential to find ways to manage it. Consider incorporating practices such as meditation, deep breathing, yoga, or spending time in nature.

5. Prioritize preventative care: Regular check-ups with your healthcare provider can help detect potential health issues early on, preventing them from becoming more severe. Stay updated on recommended health screenings, such as mammograms and other wellness checks.

Remember, self-care is not selfish; it is vital for living a happy, healthy, and fulfilling life. By prioritizing your well-being, you'll be better equipped to show up as your best self in your relationships.

What specific changes can you make in your life to prioritize your physical and mental well-being? How can investing in your own health and wellness positively impact your relationships with others, both personally and professionally?

Transition

As we've explored the significance of prioritizing our health and wellness for long-term success, we now turn our focus to the equally crucial aspect of building and nurturing healthy relationships. In the following essay, I'll share some valuable lessons I've learned about developing and maintaining meaningful connections with others. These lessons encompass effective communication, setting healthy boundaries, and practicing empathy and forgiveness. By applying these insights, we can foster more profound and fulfilling relationships and create a positive ripple effect on our overall well-being.

Yolanda Trevino

Building and Maintaining Healthy Relationships: What I Wish I Knew by 40

When it comes to relationships, there are a few valuable insights I wish I had known earlier in life. First and foremost, clear communication is essential. It's easy to assume that others can read our minds or understand what we're thinking or feeling, but that's not always the case. Learning to communicate effectively with others can help prevent misunderstandings and improve the quality of our relationships.

I also wish I had understood the importance of setting boundaries. When we fail to set boundaries with others, we can become overwhelmed and exhausted, leading to resentment and burnout. Setting boundaries is crucial for maintaining our own well-being and for building healthy relationships based on mutual respect.

Another important lesson I've learned is that it's okay to let go of toxic relationships. Sometimes, despite our best efforts, relationships can become unhealthy and even harmful. It's important to recognize when this is happening and to take action to protect ourselves.

Building and maintaining healthy relationships is vital to our personal growth and happiness. As I have experienced in my own life, the quality of our relationships can profoundly impact our overall well-being. Healthy relationships require effort and intentionality, and it's important to be discerning about who we allow into our lives.

One of the most critical lessons I've learned about healthy relationships is the significance of clear communication. Effective communication is key to preventing misunderstandings and enhancing the quality of our relationships. Moreover, setting healthy boundaries in our relationships can prevent emotional exhaustion and resentment, fostering stronger connections based on mutual respect. However, it's important to keep in mind that effective communication can only go as far as someone's understanding allows. Being mindful of this aspect can further enhance our interactions and deepen our connections with others.

Here are some practical tips for building and maintaining healthy relationships:

1. Communicate clearly and honestly: Be open and honest with your feelings and communicate your needs clearly. It's essential to listen actively to others and to seek to understand their perspective as well.

2. Set boundaries: Learn to say "no" when necessary and set limits with others in a respectful way. This can help prevent relationship fatigue and resentment, which are common consequences of overcommitment and not setting clear boundaries. In addition to saying "no" when necessary, it's important to communicate your boundaries and limits with others. This can help ensure that your needs are respected and that you're not taken advantage of.

Another essential lesson I've learned about building and maintaining healthy relationships is the value of empathy and forgiveness. When we can see things from another person's perspective and understand their feelings and needs, we can build strong, lasting connections. And when we practice forgiveness, we open ourselves up to deeper relationships with others, allowing our connections to thrive.

Finally, it's essential to be discerning about who we allow into our inner circle. Not every relationship is worth investing in, and it's important to be selective about who we allow to influence our lives. Surrounding ourselves with positive, supportive people can have a profound impact on our overall well-being and can help us cultivate healthier, more fulfilling connections with the people in our lives.

By applying these lessons and tips to our lives, we can build and maintain healthy relationships that bring us joy, fulfillment, and support. It's a lifelong journey, but one that is well worth the effort. As you reflect on your relationships, consider how you can apply these lessons to create more fulfilling connections with the people in your life. And remember, it's okay to say no to people who don't treat you well and to surround yourself with positive, supportive individuals who bring out the best in you.

In closing, I encourage you to reflect on your relationships and consider how you can apply these lessons to your life. Remember, building and maintaining healthy relationships is a lifelong journey, but one that is well worth the effort.

Who are the people in your life who bring you the most joy and fulfillment? What qualities do they possess that make those relationships so positive?

Have you ever experienced a challenging or toxic relationship? What did you learn from that experience, and how can you use that knowledge to avoid similar relationships in the future?

Transition

As you work on building and maintaining healthy relationships, it's essential to remember that everyone has their own unique challenges and struggles. By setting healthy boundaries and taking care of yourself, you can create more balanced and fulfilling relationships.

Now that we've discussed the importance of building and maintaining healthy relationships, we turn our attention to the challenges of balancing work and personal life. With the demands of modern life, it can be difficult to find time for both work and personal pursuits, leading to stress and burnout. In the following essay, we'll explore strategies for managing your time, setting priorities, and finding ways to enjoy both your professional and personal life. By learning to balance these two important aspects of your life, you can achieve greater fulfillment and satisfaction in all areas.

Balancing Work and Personal Life for Greater Fulfillment: What I Wish I Knew by 40

Balancing work and personal life is a challenge that many people face, regardless of their age or gender. Finding the right balance between the demands of work and personal life can be difficult, but it is essential for achieving greater fulfillment in life. In this essay, we will explore the importance of balancing work and personal life and provide practical tips for achieving greater balance and fulfillment.

I learned the importance of balancing work and personal life through my own experiences. When I was in my 20s, I worked long hours in unfulfilling jobs that left me feeling stressed and burnt out. I felt like I was sacrificing my personal life to prove myself in my work life, and I was struggling to find a balance.

It wasn't until my 40s that I started to reprioritize my life, making time for the things that brought me joy outside of work and found a career that I loved. I started taking walks in nature, prioritizing my health, learning new things, taking up new hobbies, and scheduling regular coffee dates with friends. As I made time for these activities, I found that my stress levels began to decrease, and my overall sense of fulfillment increased.

Finding the right balance between work and personal life can help us achieve greater fulfillment in both areas. By taking care of our personal lives, we can feel happier and more fulfilled, which can translate into greater productivity and success at work. Similarly, by focusing on our work responsibilities, we can feel more secure and confident in our personal lives.

The importance of balancing work and personal life cannot be overstated. It is a challenge that many people face and can impact our overall sense of fulfillment and well-being. In the following essay, we'll explore some strategies for managing work-life balance and overcoming challenges, so that we can emerge stronger and continue our journey towards greater fulfillment and resilience.

Here are some practical tips for achieving greater balance between work and personal life:

1. Prioritize self-care: Make self-care a priority and practice it regularly. This can include anything from taking breaks during the workday to engaging in hobbies or spending time with loved ones outside of work.

2. Learn to say no: Saying no can be difficult, but it is essential for maintaining balance and avoiding burnout. Be selective in the activities you choose to take on and don't be afraid to say no to activities that don't align with your priorities.

3. Create boundaries: Set clear boundaries between work and personal life. Avoid working during your personal time, and make sure you take breaks and vacations to recharge and relax.

4. Communicate with others: Communicate your needs and expectations with others, including your employer, colleagues, and family. Let them know when you need time off or when you need to focus on your personal life.

5. Identify your values: Identify your values and what is most important to you in life. Use this as a guide to prioritize your time and energy.

6. Find a career you love: Finding a fulfilling career can help achieve balance and fulfillment in life. Consider exploring your passions and interests to find a career that aligns with your values and provides meaning and purpose.

Remember, achieving balance is a journey, not a destination. It takes ongoing effort and intentionality to achieve. But with the right mindset and a commitment to self-care and well-being, you can achieve greater balance and fulfillment in all areas of your life.

After reading this essay, take some time to reflect on your own work-life balance. Are there areas of your life where you feel like you need to make changes to achieve greater work-life integration and fulfillment? What steps can you take to instill these changes and improve your own work-life harmony? What priorities do you need to set to achieve a better balance? Which of the tips mentioned in this essay do you find most helpful or challenging to implement? Reflect on your own experiences and start making small, intentional changes that will help you achieve a more fulfilling and balanced life.

One way to approach this is to start by identifying your values and priorities. What is most important to you in life? Is it your family, your career, your hobbies, or something else? Once you've identified your values and priorities, you can start to set goals and create a plan for achieving greater balance.

It's also important to be intentional about how you spend your time. Look for opportunities to combine work and personal life activities. For example, if you enjoy working out, consider joining a gym near your workplace so you can exercise during your lunch break. Or, if you have the flexibility to work from home, try working from a coffee shop or park to add some variety to your work routine.

Remember, finding the right balance between work and personal life is not a one-size-fits-all solution. What works for one person may not work for another. It's important to be flexible and adaptable, and to make changes as needed to achieve greater equilibrium and fulfillment.

In conclusion, balancing work and personal life is a challenge that many people face, but it's essential for achieving greater fulfillment and well-being. By setting priorities, creating boundaries, and practicing self-care, we can achieve greater balance and fulfillment in both areas of our lives. It's a journey that takes ongoing effort and intentionality, but with the right mindset and approach, we can achieve the balance we need to live a happy, healthy, and fulfilling life.

Transition

Maintaining a sense of balance is crucial not only in managing work and personal life but also in navigating the challenges that life throws our way. As we've explored the significance of achieving equilibrium in our daily lives, it's essential to acknowledge that life can be unpredictable, and we may face moments of loss and adversity. Coping with these difficult experiences requires finding a delicate balance between resilience and vulnerability. In the following essay, we'll delve into strategies for coping with loss and overcoming adversity, all while striving to maintain a sense of balance in our pursuit of greater fulfillment and well-being.

Coping with Loss and Overcoming Adversity: What I Wish I Knew by 40

When I was 30, I lost my job due to unforeseen circumstances, and I was struggling financially. I was living paycheck to paycheck and didn't know how I was going to pay my bills. I felt helpless and overwhelmed, and it was one of the lowest points in my life.

At first, I didn't know how to cope with this adversity, but I knew I needed to take action. I started looking for new job opportunities, but the job market was tough, and I wasn't having much success. I decided to focus on things that I could control, like taking care of my health and finding joy in small moments. Then, I decided to become my own boss and ventured into being a struggling entrepreneur.

As an entrepreneur in my 30s, I faced numerous setbacks, including failed business ventures, continuous financial hardship, and personal setbacks. These challenges left me feeling overwhelmed, defeated, and uncertain about the future. However, my challenges were far from over.

I found myself in a toxic relationship that had a profound impact on every aspect of my life, leaving me in ruins. The effects of this relationship were long-lasting, and for years I felt lost and broken as I struggled to recover from the damage it had caused. I had a difficult time finding a way to heal and recover from the emotional, psychological and physical trauma that I had experienced, and I turned to unhealthy coping mechanisms to escape the pain but they only brought temporary relief. Despite my efforts, healing seemed elusive, and I felt stuck in darkness, unsure of how to move forward without the proper understanding of how to begin the healing process.

Upon reaching the age of 40, I finally found a path towards transformation and healing. It became evident that self-care, the establishment of healthy boundaries, and my willingness to seek guidance were crucial in rebuilding my life. Instead of solely relying on therapy, I embarked on a journey of self-exploration, delving inward to discover the tools that resonated with me. I integrated positive experiences from my past, infusing them with newfound strategies, which ultimately empowered me to reclaim my identity and rebuild my life.

Eventually, I found success as an entrepreneur too, in career choices that I loved. Through my experiences, I learned that coping with loss and adversity is a critical part of personal growth and success. It's a process that requires patience, self-nurturing, and a willingness to take action.

Overcoming hardship is not an easy task, but it's a process that can lead to growth and healing. I learned that the key to coping with loss and adversity is to allow yourself to feel your emotions, to be kind to yourself, and to seek support when you need it. It's essential to understand that coping with loss and adversity is not a one-size-fits-all process. Everyone's journey is unique, and what works for one person may not work for another.

It's vital to find healthy coping mechanisms that work best for you, whether it's journaling, meditation, finding guidance from a life coach, or seeking professional help. One of the most important lessons I learned is that it's okay to ask for help. Seeking help is not a sign of weakness; it's a sign of strength. Whether it's a trusted friend, family member, or professional, having a support system is crucial for coping with loss and overcoming adversity.

Another lesson I learned is that it's essential to take care of yourself physically, emotionally, and mentally. It's crucial to engage in activities that bring you joy, spend time with people who uplift and support you, and make self-care a priority. These practices help to build resilience and develop the coping skills needed to overcome adversity.

It's important to remember that overcoming adversity is not a linear process. There will be ups and downs along the way, and that's okay. It's essential to give yourself grace and kindness as you navigate the journey.

At some point in our lives, we will all experience loss and adversity. Whether it's the death of a loved one, the end of a relationship, a health crisis, or a major life change, these events can be incredibly difficult to navigate. Coping with loss and adversity takes time, effort, and a willingness to confront our emotions and work through them. However, with the right mindset and strategies, it is possible to emerge from these experiences stronger and more resilient.

One of the most important lessons I learned from my own experiences is that it's okay to grieve. Losing someone or something you care about is hard, and it's natural to feel a wide range of emotions, including sadness, anger, and frustration. It's essential to give yourself the time and space to grieve in your own way and at your own pace. Allow yourself to feel the emotions that come with loss, and don't try to push your emotions away or pretend like everything is okay. Acknowledge your emotions and work through them.

Another crucial strategy for coping with loss and adversity is to find support. Coping with these challenges can be overwhelming, and it's important to have a support system in place. Surround yourself with people who care about you and are willing to listen and avoid facing it alone. Seek out support from a therapist, life coach, support group, or online community. Don't hesitate to ask for help when you need it, as seeking help is not a sign of weakness, but a sign of strength.

Are you noticing a recurring theme throughout this book? You can be confident I will continuously reiterate the significance of taking care of yourself physically, emotionally, and mentally for navigating life's challenges. Ensuring you get enough sleep, maintain a balanced diet, and engage in regular exercise are essential aspects of self-care. Moreover, participating in activities that bring joy and relaxation, such as reading, listening to music, or spending time outdoors, plays a crucial role in building resilience and developing coping skills to overcome adversity. The importance of self-care cannot be emphasized enough when facing loss and adversity.

Another lesson I learned is that focusing on what you can control is essential. When faced with loss and adversity, it's easy to feel like everything is out of your control. However, focusing on the things you can control, like your own thoughts and actions, can help you feel more empowered and less helpless. It's essential to learn how to let go of things that are outside of your control and focus on taking action on the things you can control.

It's important to remember that overcoming adversity is not a linear process. There will be ups and downs along the way, and that's okay. It's essential to give yourself grace and kindness as you navigate the journey. Recognize that healing is a process, and it's okay to take the time you need. Be patient with yourself and don't expect everything to be resolved overnight.

Coping with loss and overcoming adversity is a difficult but necessary part of life. It's a process that can lead to growth, self-discovery, and resilience. Remember to be kind to yourself, seek support when you need it, and engage in activities that promote self-care. With the right mindset and support, you can overcome adversity and find strength in the face of loss. Finally, remember that you're not alone, and there is always hope for a better tomorrow.

Take some time now to reflect on your own experiences and what you can do to build resilience and overcome adversity. Remember, there is no right or wrong way to cope with loss and adversity. What matters most is finding healthy ways to manage your emotions and move forward.

What coping mechanisms have worked for you in the past when dealing with loss or adversity? In what ways have your experiences with loss or adversity shaped who you are today?

Transition

Having the ability to overcome adversity and find strength within yourself is a powerful tool to have when it comes to living an authentic life. After learning how to overcome adversity and cope with loss, we are ready to dive deeper into personal growth and self-discovery. Embracing our true selves and finding our voice is an essential step on this journey. In this next essay, we'll explore the importance of self-acceptance, self-expression, and how to navigate roadblocks that stand in the way of our authentic selves. Let's continue on this journey of growth and self-discovery.

Embracing Your Authentic Self and Finding Your Voice: What I Wish I Knew By 40

As you're aware, for much of my career before I began working for myself, I worked in corporate settings where I felt pressured to conform to a conservative and stifling culture. I tried to fit into a mold that didn't fit me, which made me feel unfulfilled and unhappy. To make matters worse, I found myself in relationships that weren't authentic, accepting people into my life who didn't share my values and left me feeling drained and unsupported and in some cases, in ruins.

Dealing with office politics and encountering behavior reminiscent of high school mean girls added to the complexity of these challenges. The toxic dynamics of such environments further fueled my desire to seek a more balanced and authentic life. Through my journey of self-discovery and healing, I recognized the immense value of self-care. By prioritizing my well-being and practicing self-compassion, I gradually learned to protect myself from the negative influences of these settings.

Breaking free from the constraints of an unsatisfying corporate culture and aligning my life with my authentic values and aspirations allowed me to find my voice and express my true self. This book delves into the significance of this journey, not only during life's major adversities but also in navigating the subtler, yet equally impactful, challenges encountered in professional and social settings. Finding your voice becomes a guiding principle for resilience, personal growth, and fulfillment, allowing you to thrive and maintain your sense of self in any environment.

It wasn't until I started setting boundaries for myself and embracing my authenticity that I began to feel more fulfilled and empowered. Learning to say "no" to things that didn't align with my values and taking risks to pursue my passions gave me the confidence to speak up and be myself. Despite the fact that some people rejected or abandoned me when I embraced my true self, and others tried to take advantage of me, I stood up for myself and refused to let their judgment or anyone else's hold me back.

In reflecting on my own journey towards embracing my authentic self and finding my voice, here are some things I wish I had known by the time I turned 40:

1. Embrace your uniqueness: We are all different, and that's what makes us special. Don't try to change yourself to fit into

someone else's mold. Embrace your unique qualities, whether they are physical, personality traits, or skills.

2. Listen to your inner voice: Your intuition is always trying to guide you in the right direction. Listen to it and trust it, even if it's telling you to do something that scares you.

3. Identify your values: Knowing what's most important to you can help you make decisions that align with your true self. Take some time to identify your values and make sure your actions and decisions reflect them.

4. Learn to say "no": Saying "no" can be difficult, especially if you're used to saying "yes" to everything. But it's important to set boundaries and prioritize your own needs. Saying "no" can be empowering and help you take control of your life, especially when there are those that are used to taking advantage of or manipulating you.

5. Take risks: Embracing your authentic self and finding your voice can be scary. It means putting yourself out there and taking risks. But taking risks is what allows us to grow and discover our true potential.

6. Surround yourself with supportive people: Finding your voice and embracing your authentic self is much easier when you have a supportive network of people around you. Seek out

people who uplift and encourage you, and avoid those who bring you down.

7. Practice self-care: Taking care of yourself is crucial when trying to embrace your authentic self and find your voice. Make time for self-care activities that help you relax, whether it's meditation, yoga, or spending time outdoors.

8. Embrace imperfection: We are all imperfect, and that's okay. Embrace your flaws and use them to your advantage. Your imperfections make you unique and special and are an essential part of your authentic self and voice.

The journey towards embracing your authentic self and finding your voice is ongoing. It's never too late to start, and every step you take towards your true self is a step towards living a more fulfilling and satisfying life.

Here are some additional ideas to expand on the ways to embrace your authentic self and find your voice:

1. Practice self-reflection: Take time to reflect on your thoughts, feelings, and experiences. Self-reflection can help you gain a deeper understanding of yourself and what's important to you.

2. Be true to yourself: When making decisions, consider what you really want, rather than what others want for you. It's important to prioritize your own needs and desires, and to be true to yourself.

3. Identify your strengths and weaknesses: Knowing your strengths and weaknesses can help you make decisions that align with your natural abilities and skills, and help you overcome challenges and areas for growth.

4. Overcome fear: Fear can hold you back from embracing your authentic self and finding your voice. Identify the fears that are holding you back, and work to overcome them. Remember, taking risks is what allows us to grow and discover our true potential.

5. Set goals and create a plan: Setting goals and creating a plan can help you stay focused and motivated as you work towards embracing your authentic self and finding your voice. Consider what steps you can take to achieve your goals, and break them down into smaller, more manageable tasks.

6. Seek support: Surround yourself with people who support and encourage you. Seek out mentors, coaches, or counselors who can help you along your journey.

7. Take action: Embracing your authentic self and finding your voice requires action. Start taking small steps towards your goals, and keep pushing yourself out of your comfort zone.

8. Cultivate self-compassion: Treat yourself with kindness and compassion, especially when you make mistakes or experience setbacks. Embracing your authentic self is a

journey, and it's important to be patient and kind with yourself along the way.

9. Explore your passions: Take the time to explore what you truly enjoy and what brings you joy. This can help you identify your passions and values, which can guide you towards a more fulfilling life.

10. Express yourself creatively: Engage in creative activities like writing, drawing, or painting. These activities can help you connect with your emotions and express yourself in new and unique ways.

11. Take care of your physical health: Your physical health can have a significant impact on your mental and emotional well-being. Taking care of your body through exercise, nutrition, and sleep can help you feel more energized, focused, and confident.

After reading about embracing your authentic self and finding your voice, take some time to reflect on your own journey towards self-discovery and embracing who you truly are. In what ways have you tried to fit into other people's expectations of who you should be, and how has that affected your sense of self? What steps can you take to embrace your authentic self and live in alignment with your true values and passions? Remember, finding your voice is about expressing your true self confidently, and this process may involve continuous growth and self-exploration.

Remember that embracing your authentic self and finding your voice is a journey unique to each individual. It requires self-reflection, patience, and effort, but the result is a more fulfilling and satisfying life. Start by taking small steps towards self-discovery and self-acceptance, and be kind and compassionate with yourself along the way. In time you will begin to discover your true self, find your voice, and live a more fulfilling life.

Transition

Now that we've explored how to embrace your authentic self and find your voice, let's shift our focus to an important aspect of life: finances. In the next essay, we'll share some tips on managing your finances and planning for the future. We'll cover topics such as creating a budget, saving for emergencies and retirement, and managing debt. Taking control of your finances can provide a sense of security and peace of mind, so let's dive in and learn how to better manage our money.

Tips for Managing Finances and Planning for the Future: What I Wish I Knew by 40

There are some valuable lessons to be learned from our financial experiences that can help us build a better financial future for ourselves. Personal struggles can impact our financial behavior and make managing finances more challenging. For me, dealing with the aftermath of a traumatic event led me down a path of overspending, debt, and financial stress. It took years for me to realize that my financial struggles were related to the trauma I had experienced, and I had to make difficult choices, such as moving into living situations that I didn't enjoy, to get by. Eventually, I was able to turn things around and learned important lessons about managing finances.

As we go through life, we learn valuable lessons that shape who we are today. When it comes to finances, it's no different. We all make mistakes and face financial struggles along the way. However, these experiences can teach us important lessons that we can use to build a better financial future for ourselves. Here are some of the lessons I've learned about managing finances that I wish I knew by the time I was 40.

Create a Budget and Stick to It

Creating a budget is crucial when managing finances. It helps you track your income and expenses and assists in managing your money. I used to be a stickler for writing everything down in my checkbook and keeping a daily tab total running. However, after a traumatic experience at the age of 19, I started to develop a problem with managing my money. As a means to cope, I became a major shopaholic, which caused me to incur significant debt. I realized years later that this was related to my trauma. So, creating a budget is not just about keeping track of money, but it can also help you manage any emotional issues that may be impacting your finances.

Avoid Debt When Possible

Debt can be a significant burden that affects your financial health and limits your financial freedom. While some forms of debt, such as a mortgage or a car loan, may be necessary, it's important to avoid high-interest debt, such as credit cards, whenever possible. If you do have debt, make sure to prioritize paying it off as soon as possible. I struggled with debt for many years, and it wasn't until I made a conscious effort to avoid it that I was able to start making progress.

Build an Emergency Fund

Life is unpredictable, and unexpected expenses can arise at any time. To avoid going into debt or feeling financial stress when emergencies occur, it's important to build an emergency fund. This should be a separate savings account where you set aside money for unexpected expenses, such as car repairs or medical bills. Aim to have at least three to six months' worth of living expenses saved in your emergency fund. Building an emergency fund was something I wish I had started earlier in life, as it would have saved me from many financial emergencies.

Save for Retirement

It's never too early or too late to start saving for retirement. The earlier you start, the more time your money has to grow, but even if you're starting later in life, it's still important to save as much as you can. Take advantage of employer-sponsored retirement plans, such as 401(k) plans, and contribute as much as you can afford. If you don't have access to a retirement plan through work, consider opening an Individual Retirement Account (IRA). I regret not starting to save for retirement earlier, as it would have given me more financial security in my later years.

Invest in Yourself

Investing in yourself is one of the most important investments you can make. This can take many forms, such as education or training that can lead to higher-paying job opportunities, going into business for yourself, or even just taking care of your physical and mental health. When you invest in yourself, you're increasing your potential to earn more money and improve your financial situation. Investing in myself helped me gain the confidence to take control of my finances and make better financial decisions.

Don't Compare Yourself to Others

Comparing yourself to others is a surefire way to feel dissatisfied with your financial situation. Everyone's financial journey is different, and it's important to focus on your own goals and progress. Instead of comparing yourself to others, set your own financial goals and work towards them at your own pace. It's easy to feel inadequate when comparing yourself to others, especially when it comes to finances. However, it's essential to remember that everyone's financial journey is unique, and it's important to focus on your own progress rather than comparing yourself to others. When setting financial goals, make sure they're realistic and tailored to your own situation, rather than trying to match someone else's accomplishments.

Seek Expert Financial Guidance When Necessary

Managing finances can be a daunting task, and it's okay to seek out the help of an expert when necessary. A financial advisor or planner can help you create a personalized financial plan and offer advice on how to achieve your goals. It's important to find a professional you trust and feel comfortable working with. They can help you make sense of complex financial concepts and develop strategies to improve your financial situation.

In conclusion, managing finances is a crucial skill that can lead to a more secure and fulfilling future. By creating a budget, avoiding high-interest debt, building an emergency fund, saving for retirement, investing in yourself, not comparing yourself to others, and seeking professional help when necessary, you can take control of your financial situation and build a better financial future. These are the lessons that I wish I knew by the time I was 40, but they are still relevant to me today.

At the end of the essay, "Tips for Managing Finances and Planning for the Future," take a moment to reflect on your own financial situation and the steps you can take to achieve your goals. Consider the following questions:

- What are my short-term and long-term financial goals?

- What are some specific steps I can take to achieve those goals?

Remember, taking control of your finances is an ongoing process, and it's never too late to start. Whether it's creating a budget, seeking financial advice, or exploring new sources of income, every step you take towards financial stability is a step in the right direction. By following these tips and staying committed to your financial goals, you can build a better financial future for yourself and your loved ones.

Transition

As we've seen, managing finances can indeed be an intimidating and overwhelming task that demands effort, planning, and self-reflection. From creating a budget to investing in oneself and seeking professional guidance, the steps taken to handle finances can significantly impact one's financial health and overall well-being. Having delved into the essential aspects of managing finances and planning for a secure future, we now shift our focus to another vital facet of life: finding joy and meaning in our everyday experiences.

Finding Joy and Meaning in Everyday Life: What I Wish I Knew by 40

As I experienced a life-altering and traumatic event in my 30s, I found myself trapped in a decade-long depressive episode, which left my life seemingly dull and devoid of joy and excitement. It felt as if there was no escape from the darkness that engulfed me, and I began to believe the frightening and untrue notion that my life had come to an end. During this time, I had difficulty being optimistic and seeing opportunities in everything and everywhere. Part of the struggle came from certain individuals in my life who caused chaos and distress, significantly adding to the challenges I was facing after I had lost my job. However, through relentless efforts to improve and armed with the right tools and mindset, I was able to overcome the sources of my distress, which lay at the root of my constant depressive episodes. Finally, after many years of perseverance, I began to appreciate the joy and beauty in life, even in the smallest things that I had overlooked before. I learned to see life as vibrant, choosing to enjoy the beautiful flowers that I used to ignore and taking in the wonder they brought to the world. I discovered a new appreciation for whole natural foods and cultivated a mindset of gratitude by following the tips I'm sharing in this essay and throughout the book. The beauty and innocence in wildlife and nature are now a daily source of joy and wonder. I no longer take them for granted but instead, I stop, breathe, and quiet my mind to see the beauty in everything.

Life is a journey, and discovering joy and meaning in everyday experiences is a crucial aspect of that voyage. Allow me to share the valuable insights I've gained on my own path to finding joy and meaning in life, helping you avoid enduring years of anguish searching for answers on how to recapture your joy and live life to the fullest:

1. Practice gratitude: One of the most effective ways to find joy and meaning in everyday life is to practice gratitude. Take a moment each day to reflect on the things you're grateful for, whether it's your health, your relationships, or the opportunities that have come your way. Focusing on what you have, rather than what you lack, can help shift your mindset and lead to greater happiness.

2. Make time for what you enjoy: It's important to make time for the things you enjoy, whether it's reading, writing, painting, or spending time with loved ones. Make it a priority to schedule time for these activities, even if it's just for a few minutes each

day. Doing what you love can help you feel more fulfilled and bring joy to your everyday life.

3. Connect with others: We are social beings, and it's important to connect with others to find joy and meaning in everyday life. Whether it's spending time with friends, joining a club or organization, or volunteering in your community, connecting with others can help you feel more fulfilled and bring purpose to your daily routine.

4. Find beauty in the ordinary: There is beauty all around us, even in the most ordinary of things. Take a moment to appreciate the sunrise, the sound of birds singing, the innocence of children or the smell of freshly brewed coffee. Finding beauty in the ordinary can help you appreciate the little things in life, capture fleeting moments, and bring joy to your everyday routine.

5. Challenge yourself: Sometimes it can be easy to get stuck in a routine and lose the sense of excitement and meaning in our lives. Challenge yourself to try something new, whether it's learning a new skill, attending a networking function, taking up a new hobby, or traveling to a new place. Stepping outside of your comfort zone can help you grow as a person and find new sources of joy and meaning in your life.

6. Practice mindfulness: Mindfulness is the practice of being present and fully engaged in the moment. It can help us

appreciate the small things in life and find joy and meaning in everyday experiences. Practice mindfulness by focusing on your breath, noticing your surroundings, or simply taking a moment to be still and present.

7. Give back to others: Helping others can be a powerful source of joy and meaning in our lives. Whether it's volunteering in your community, donating to charity, or simply offering a kind word to someone in need, giving back can help you feel more connected to others and bring a sense of purpose to your life.

8. By practicing these tips, you can find joy and meaning in everyday life, even in the most mundane of days. Remember, life is a journey, and it's up to you to make the most of it.

Remembering to find joy and meaning in everyday life can sometimes be challenging. Take a moment to reflect on what brings you joy and meaning in your life as you consider these questions:

1. What activities bring you joy and make you feel fulfilled?

2. How can you incorporate more of these activities into your daily life?

Transition

As you learn to cultivate joy in your everyday life, you'll come to recognize that with age often comes a desire to seek out more purpose and fulfillment in our careers. As we grow and change, our professional aspirations may shift, leading us to explore new opportunities and career paths. For some, this can be an exciting time of self-discovery, but for others, it can be a daunting and uncertain process. In the next section, we will explore the challenges and opportunities that come with navigating career changes and finding your purpose. Whether you're just starting out in your career or considering a change later in life, these tips and insights can help guide you towards a more fulfilling and purposeful professional journey. So, let's dive in and explore tips for navigating career changes and finding your purpose, helping you identify your passions and set goals for the future.

Navigating Career Changes and Finding Your Purpose: What I Wish I Knew by 40

Throughout my work-life journey, I have experienced multiple major career changes that have challenged me to navigate new paths and find my true purpose. I experienced a major turning point in my career when I lost my job at 30. The experience of being laid off forced me to reassess my career path and make important decisions about my future.

At first, the idea of starting my own business was daunting and filled me with anxiety. I had spent most of my professional life in a rigid corporate environment where creativity and self-expression were discouraged, and I worried that I wouldn't be able to handle the uncertainty and risk that came with entrepreneurship. But I knew deep down that I wanted something more fulfilling and meaningful out of my career, and so I took the leap and started my own company. It was a challenging journey filled with ups and downs, as I had to learn how to navigate a whole new world of entrepreneurship. However, I quickly discovered that starting my own business was the best decision I ever made. It allowed me to be my own boss, follow my passion, and create something of my own that was both personally and professionally fulfilling.

Over the next 15 years, I continued to grow and evolve as an entrepreneur. However, my journey was not without its share of challenges. I faced many ups and downs, and then, during the pandemic, when the world was shutting down and businesses were struggling to survive, I was confronted with one of the most formidable obstacles.

The pandemic brought unprecedented uncertainty, and the future of my business, Microhair Aesthetics, seemed precarious. Yet, I was determined to rise to the occasion. Despite the external circumstances beyond my control, I persevered through these difficult times, working tirelessly to overcome the obstacles that came my way. It wasn't an effortless endeavor, but through resilience and determination, I managed to pivot my business and adapt to the new reality.

In the face of the pandemic's impact on the beauty and wellness industry, I made the bold decision to shift my focus. What initially began as a permanent cosmetics service transformed into a multi-faceted online platform. I ventured into selling skin care, hair care and supplement products, which not only addressed the evolving needs of my clients but also expanded my business's reach.

As my business took on a new direction, I embraced the opportunity to diversify my offerings further. I became an author and I launched an online life coaching program called Evolutionary Body System. The program delves deep into the realms of personal growth and self-discovery, empowering individuals from the inside out, and igniting profound transformations in their lives. It provides valuable insights to address the weight they carry from life's challenges and traumas, guiding them towards healing and understanding to overcome these obstacles that have been buried within. The Evolutionary Body System is a journey of inner transformation, allowing individuals to shed the burdens of the past and embrace a renewed sense of self, ultimately leading to a fulfilling and purposeful life.

Though the journey has been challenging, this pivot has allowed me to discover new horizons and tap into the ever-expanding digital landscape. With the Evolutionary Body System, I can now reach and help individuals beyond the confines of a physical location, making a profound impact on lives far and wide. This book itself is a byproduct of that coaching program, offering readers a glimpse of how to transform themselves from within, empowering them to embrace their imperfections and embark on their journey of growth and self-acceptance.

Through my career changes and experiences as an entrepreneur, I have learned the importance of staying true to my values, being open to new opportunities and learning experiences, and seeking out mentors and support to help me navigate the challenges along the way.

Now, as we go through life, it's common to find ourselves in a state of transition, especially when it comes to our careers. We may feel the need to pivot, whether that's due to a lack of fulfillment, a desire for a new challenge, or external circumstances like a job loss or industry changes. But making a career change can be intimidating, especially when we're not sure what our purpose is or what we want to do next. Let's explore some tips and lessons I learned by 40 and continue to learn, for navigating career changes and finding your purpose.

Tips and Lessons

Assess Your Values and Interests:

When considering a career change, it's important to start by assessing your values and interests. These are the things that bring you the most joy and fulfillment in life and can help guide you towards a purposeful career. Start by asking yourself questions like:

- What motivates and inspires me?
- What are my unique talents and strengths?
- What are my core values?
- What activities or hobbies do I enjoy?

Taking the time to answer these questions can help you identify potential career paths that align with your passions and purpose.

Network and Seek Out Informational Interviews:

Once you have a general idea of your values and interests, it's important to network and seek out informational interviews with professionals in fields that interest you. This can help you get a better sense of what a particular job or industry is really like and help you decide if it's a good fit for you. Be proactive in reaching out to people in your network or on LinkedIn and ask if they would be willing to have a conversation with you. Come prepared with thoughtful questions and be open to learning from their experiences.

Embrace the Process of Growth and Evolution:

This is essential when navigating career changes and finding your purpose. It's not a linear journey, and there will be moments of uncertainty, setbacks, and self-doubt along the way. These experiences can be worrisome, chaotic, and full of twists and turns, but they're all part of the journey. Instead of being discouraged by the inevitable bumps in the road, use them as opportunities to reflect on what you've learned and adjust your course. Embracing this process of growth and evolution can help you stay motivated and focused on your ultimate goal of finding a fulfilling and purposeful career.

Don't be Afraid to Take Risks:

When making a career change, it's important to be willing to take risks. This may mean stepping outside of your comfort zone, taking on a new challenge, or even making a financial investment in your education or training. It can be scary to take a leap of faith, but it's often necessary to make meaningful progress in your career and find your purpose. Be open to new possibilities and don't be afraid to take calculated risks.

Get Support and Guidance:

Making a career change can be a challenging and isolating experience, but it doesn't have to be. Seek out support and guidance from friends, family, or a career coach. Having a sounding board can help you work through the tough decisions and stay motivated when the going gets tough. A career coach can offer additional guidance and support, help you clarify your values and goals, and provide actionable steps to help you achieve them.

Keep an Open Mind and Be Willing to Learn:

Navigating career changes and finding your purpose is an ongoing process, and it's important to keep an open mind and be willing to learn. This means being open to feedback, seeking out new experiences, and learning new skills. It also means being open to new possibilities and opportunities that may present themselves along the way.

It's never too late to learn something new or try a new career path. In fact, many successful people have made multiple career changes throughout their lives. Don't be afraid to try something new and learn as much as you can along the way. You never know where it may lead you.

Seek Out Mentors and Role Models:

Having mentors and role models can be invaluable when it comes to navigating career changes and finding your purpose. These individuals can provide guidance, support, and inspiration as you explore new opportunities and pursue your goals. Look for individuals in your field who have achieved success and are willing to share their knowledge and experience with you. Connect with them, ask for advice, and learn from their successes and failures.

Network and Build Relationships:

Networking is an important part of navigating career changes and finding your purpose. Building relationships with others in your field can open up new opportunities, provide valuable insights, and give you access to new resources and information.

Attend networking events, join professional organizations, and connect with others in your field through social media and other online platforms. Be proactive in building relationships and seek out opportunities to connect with others.

Stay Flexible and Adapt to Change:

The world of work is constantly evolving, and it's important to stay flexible and adapt to change as you navigate your career and find your purpose. This means being open to new technologies, new ideas, and new ways of working. It also means being willing to take risks, try new things, and pivot when necessary. Don't be afraid to make changes and take bold steps in pursuit of your goals.

Embrace the Journey:

Navigating career changes and finding your purpose is a journey, and it's important to embrace the process and enjoy the ride. It may not always be easy, and there may be setbacks and challenges along the way. But by staying focused, learning from your experiences, and staying true to your values and passions, you can find fulfillment and purpose in your work.

Remember that finding your purpose is not a one-time event. It's an ongoing process that requires reflection, learning, and adaptation. By staying open, seeking out support and guidance, and staying true to yourself, you can navigate career changes and find your purpose in life.

Navigating career changes and finding your purpose is a journey that requires self-reflection, self-awareness, and a willingness to take risks. But by staying true to yourself and following your passions, you can find fulfillment and purpose in your work. Keep in mind that your purpose may change over time as you grow and evolve as a person, and that's okay. Embrace the journey and trust in yourself to make the right decisions for your career and life.

In conclusion, navigating career changes and finding your purpose is a journey that can be challenging but also incredibly rewarding. By assessing your values and interests, networking and seeking out guidance, staying open to new possibilities, and taking care of yourself, you can find a fulfilling and purposeful career that aligns with your passions and values. Remember to embrace the journey and trust in yourself to make the right decisions for your career and life.

Before you go, take some time to reflect on your career journey thus far. Consider the experiences that have led you to where you are today, and the values and passions that have driven you along the way. Then, ponder the following questions:

1. What are some of the most meaningful experiences you've had in your career, and how have they shaped your perspective?

2. How can you align your work with your values and passions, and use your skills to make a positive impact in the world?

Transition

As we journey through life, we inevitably encounter a myriad of challenges, ranging from navigating career changes and discovering our purpose to coping with setbacks and uncertainties. Among these obstacles, one of the most formidable can be the unyielding pressure to achieve perfection—to have every aspect of our lives perfectly in order, free from any missteps or errors. In the upcoming essay, we will delve into invaluable tips and lessons that shed light on how to release the grip of perfectionism and embrace the beauty of imperfection as a powerful catalyst for growth and self-discovery. Here, I offer the wisdom I gained when it comes to letting go of perfectionism.

Letting Go of Perfectionism: What I Wish I Knew by 40

For most of my life, I struggled with the need to be perfect. I didn't like to ask for help, because I didn't want to appear vulnerable or incompetent. This led me to cultivate a mindset of self-reliance and control, where I believed that I had to do everything on my own. I thought that being perfect would protect me from criticism, judgment, and failure, and that people would like me more if I didn't show any weaknesses. But the truth was, I was making my own feelings of inadequacy worse by not allowing myself to learn and grow.

As I got older, I realized that being a perfectionist was hindering my personal and professional growth. I was constantly anxious and stressed, always worried that I wasn't doing enough or that I would make a mistake. I was setting unrealistic expectations for myself, and when I inevitably fell short, I would beat myself up for it. I had to let go of my fear of failure and embrace my imperfections.

This process was challenging, but it brought positive changes to my life. Letting go of perfectionism allowed me to feel free in my choices and accept failures as part of life and my career. For example, as a public speaker, I used to believe that I had to be perfect when speaking in public and that any mistake would be a failure. This caused me to feel incredibly anxious before speaking engagements and made me hesitant to take on new opportunities. However, by letting go of my perfectionism and embracing imperfection, I was able to shift my focus to the message and the experience, rather than worrying about being flawless. This allowed me to be more authentic, connect better with my audience, and feel more fulfilled by the experience.

Embracing imperfection is an ongoing process, but it has allowed me to appreciate the journey and be more present in the moment. It has allowed me to take on new challenges with a growth mindset and to find joy in the learning process. By letting go of perfectionism, I have been able to pursue my passions more fully and to enjoy life on my own terms.

As we grow older, we realize that life is not always easy, and it doesn't always go as planned. We face challenges, obstacles, and failures that can leave us feeling discouraged and frustrated. For many of us, the need for perfectionism becomes a way of coping with the uncertainty and chaos of life. We believe that if we can control every aspect of our lives and be perfect, we can avoid the pain of failure and disappointment. I have learned that perfectionism is not a solution; it is a problem. It can lead to stress, anxiety, and burnout, and it can prevent us from living a fulfilling life and even be counterproductive to achieving one's goals.

Perfectionism is often viewed as a desirable trait, particularly among high-achievers. However, while striving for excellence can lead to success, the pursuit of perfection can often lead to negative consequences. It can cause stress, anxiety, and self-criticism.

For many people, perfectionism is a habit that is difficult to break, and it can take a toll on physical, emotional, and mental health. As a recovering perfectionist, I have come to understand how perfectionism can lead to self-criticism, anxiety, and burnout. I spent a large part of my life trying to be perfect in everything I did, from my career to personal relationships. I held myself to high standards and always pushed myself to do better, but I often found myself feeling overwhelmed and stressed. It was only when I started to let go of the need to be perfect that I started to find balance and inner peace.

Letting go of perfectionism is an essential life skill that can lead to greater happiness, fulfillment, and success. It is something that I wish I knew by the time I was 40, but it is never too late to start. By embracing imperfection, setting realistic goals, and being kinder to ourselves, we can learn to let go of the need to be perfect and live a more fulfilling life.

One of the most important things I have learned about letting go of perfectionism is that it is not about settling for mediocrity or giving up on excellence. Instead, it is about recognizing that there is a difference between striving for excellence and striving for perfection. While perfection is an unattainable goal, excellence is a standard that we can aspire to without sacrificing our well-being.

Another crucial aspect of letting go of perfectionism is learning to embrace imperfection. Accepting that we are not perfect, and that mistakes and failures are an inevitable part of life, can help us to become more resilient and develop a growth mindset. It is only by making mistakes and learning from them that we can grow and become better versions of ourselves.

There are many practical steps we can take to let go of perfectionism. One important step is to set realistic expectations and goals for ourselves. It is essential to recognize our limitations and not overburden ourselves with unrealistic expectations. It is also helpful to reframe our self-talk to be more positive and encouraging. Instead of being self-critical, we can learn to be more self-compassionate and forgiving.

In addition, practicing mindfulness and self-care can help us to let go of perfectionism. By becoming more aware of our thoughts and emotions, we can learn to manage stress and anxiety better. We can also develop healthier coping mechanisms, such as exercise, meditation, or spending time with loved ones. Engaging in activities that bring us joy and relaxation can help us let go of our need for perfection and focus on the present moment. Additionally, taking care of our physical health, such as getting enough sleep and eating a balanced diet, can also help us manage stress and anxiety. When we prioritize our physical health, we are better equipped to handle life's challenges, and we are more resilient in the face of adversity.

In conclusion, letting go of perfectionism is not an overnight process, and it can take time and practice to develop a healthier mindset. However, it is a worthwhile journey that can lead to greater happiness, fulfillment, and success. By embracing imperfection, setting realistic goals, and being kinder to ourselves, we can learn to let go of the need to be perfect and live a more fulfilling life. Remember, we are all human, and it is okay to make mistakes and learn from them. Letting go of perfectionism can allow us to experience more joy and freedom in life, to appreciate our successes, and to have more compassion for ourselves and others.

As we go through life, many of us struggle with the pressure of perfectionism. We think we need to have everything figured out and be the best at everything we do, but that kind of thinking can hold us back and prevent us from truly enjoying our lives. In this essay, I shared what I learned about letting go of perfectionism and embracing imperfection. I hope this essay has encouraged you to let go of your own perfectionist tendencies and embrace your unique path.

As you reflect on what you've read, consider these questions:

1. What are some areas of your life where you tend to be a perfectionist? How has that impacted you?

2. How can you start to let go of perfectionism and embrace imperfection in your life?

Remember that letting go of perfectionism is a journey, not a destination. Be patient and compassionate with yourself as you work on developing a healthier mindset. With time and practice, you can learn to embrace imperfection and live a more fulfilling life.

Transition

Given the insightful exploration of letting go of perfectionism in the previous essay, it's crucial to recognize that the pursuit of perfection often stems from a fear of failure or disappointment. As we strive for perfection, we attempt to gain control over every aspect of our lives to avoid potential pain or judgment. However, this mindset can lead to negative consequences, including stress, anxiety, and burnout. As I approach my 50s, I have come to understand the significance of letting go of perfectionism and embracing imperfection. Nevertheless, I've also realized that mastering the art of overcoming fear is another essential life skill that can profoundly impact our journey. In the forthcoming section, I will share what I wish I knew by 40 about overcoming fear and how it can unlock a more fulfilling and successful life.

Overcoming Fear: What I Wish I Knew by 40

Fear is a natural emotion that can both protect and hinder us in living a fulfilling life. As someone who has encountered her fair share of fears, I can attest to the importance of learning to overcome them as a vital life skill. Throughout my journey, fear often acted as a barrier, causing me to hold back from pursuing my dreams and hindering me from embracing the life I truly desired. It even led me to spend precious years in toxic relationships, taking time to heal from their impact.

It wasn't until I reached my 40s that I began to take control of my life and confront my fears. Overcoming fear required considerable self-reflection, self-awareness, and courage. Rather than aiming to be completely fearless, I learned that overcoming fear meant acknowledging it and taking action despite feeling afraid. Stepping out of my comfort zones and embracing risks, even when unsure of the outcome, became pivotal in my journey. Understanding that fear is a natural emotion and need not dictate my decisions was liberating.

In my experience, identifying my fears and taking small steps were crucial components of overcoming them. I embarked on a journey of self-discovery, examining the aspects of life that triggered anxiety and fear within me. By setting realistic, achievable goals, I gradually built confidence and gained momentum in confronting my fears. Additionally, challenging negative thoughts and beliefs was instrumental in breaking free from the shackles of fear. Many of our fears are rooted in irrational thoughts, and replacing them with positive, realistic beliefs was transformative.

Another essential aspect of my fear-conquering journey was practicing self-care. Taking care of my well-being became essential in facing fear. Prioritizing rest, maintaining a healthy diet, and engaging in regular exercise reduced my stress and anxiety, allowing me to approach fear with greater resilience. Seeking support from friends, family, and professionals was also invaluable. Overcoming fear can be daunting, but having a support system made the journey more manageable.

Taking action was the ultimate key to overcoming fear. While fear may persist, taking steps forward despite its presence empowers us to reclaim control of our lives. Starting with small, manageable steps and gradually pushing the boundaries of my comfort zone, I realized that I could grow and achieve beyond what I once thought possible. Taking action became synonymous with taking charge of my life, not letting fear hold me back.

While fear can indeed be a hindrance, I have come to understand that it need not dictate our paths. By identifying our fears, taking small steps, challenging negative thoughts, practicing self-care, seeking support, and taking action, we can conquer our fears and embrace a life of fulfillment. Embracing our fears and using them as stepping stones toward growth can lead to transformative change.

As you reflect on your life, consider the fears that may have held you back in the past. Examine the negative thoughts and beliefs that limit your potential. Find the courage to challenge them and nurture your self-confidence. In the journey of overcoming fear, remember that it's never too late to start, and with dedication, perseverance, and a willingness to take risks, you can achieve what you once thought impossible.

Recognize that conquering fear is an ongoing process that requires time and effort. Yet, the rewards of overcoming fear are immeasurable. Embrace a life filled with purpose and confidence, empowering you to pursue your passions and dreams with renewed vigor.

As you progress in conquering your fears, practice self-compassion and patience. Celebrate even the smallest successes along the way. Moreover, don't hesitate to seek support from friends, family, or professionals when needed. Embrace the journey of overcoming fear as an opportunity for growth and self-discovery.

In summary, fear is a natural and normal emotion that can hinder us from living a fulfilling life. However, by acknowledging our fears, taking small steps, challenging negative thoughts, practicing self-care, and taking action, we can overcome fear's grasp and embrace the life we desire. It's never too late to start this transformative journey, and with dedication and resilience, we can achieve what once seemed beyond our reach.

As you contemplate your own fears, consider the negative thoughts and beliefs that may be holding you back. Identify areas where you can take small steps and build your confidence. Cultivate self-care as you face your fears, and don't hesitate to seek support from those around you. Remember, fear is not a barrier that needs to imprison you; it can be the catalyst for growth and empowerment. Embrace your fears, confront them with courage, and take action towards the life you truly want.

Now, take a moment to reflect on your own life, think about some of the fears that have held you back. What are some of the negative thoughts and beliefs that you have about yourself or your abilities? What small steps can you take to challenge those thoughts and build your confidence? How can you take care of yourself and seek support when facing your fears? What is one action you can take today to move towards your goals, even if it scares you?

Transition

As you work on overcoming your fears and taking action towards your goals, effective communication can be a crucial tool to help you connect with others, build strong relationships, and achieve success. In "The Importance of Communication: What I Wish I Knew By 40," you'll discover key strategies for expressing yourself assertively, listening actively, and building meaningful connections with those around you. Whether you're looking to improve your personal or professional relationships, this essay will provide valuable insights and techniques to help you communicate more effectively and achieve your goals.

The Importance of Communication: What I Wish I Knew by 40

Effective communication is a cornerstone of human interaction, often overlooked, yet it plays a pivotal role in creating strong and meaningful relationships, both on personal and professional fronts. Reflecting on my life, I have come to realize the paramount importance of cultivating effective communication skills from an early age. During my formative years, I encountered challenges in honing my ability to express my thoughts, emotions, and opinions with clarity and confidence.

As I embarked on the journey through my 40s, I realized that communication is not merely a means of exchanging words but a transformative force that can shape the course of one's life. My inability to convey my emotions effectively in the past led to misunderstandings and frustrations. However, with a renewed commitment to self-improvement, I dedicated myself to learning and practicing effective communication, active listening, and conflict resolution. This transformational process enabled me to build stronger relationships and navigate difficult situations with newfound ease.

Effective communication serves as the bridge that connects individuals, fostering understanding, respect, and trust. By articulating our needs, feelings, and opinions in a respectful and assertive manner, we create an environment where misunderstandings and conflicts are minimized, and connections with others are strengthened. Emphasizing the importance of empathy, I learned to understand and validate the perspectives and emotions of others, leading to more compassionate and meaningful interactions. Stepping into their shoes, I built stronger bonds, nurturing a sense of understanding and support.

Listening actively, often an overlooked aspect of communication, proved to be a critical skill. By becoming an attentive listener, I honed the ability to interpret not only the words but also the tone and body language of others. This deeper level of engagement helped me avoid misunderstandings and foster more profound connections. Additionally, I recognized the significance of non-verbal communication – the power of body language, eye contact, and facial expressions – which can convey emotions and messages more effectively than words alone. Being mindful of both my own non-verbal cues and interpreting those of others further enhanced my overall communication skills.

Conflict resolution, closely related to effective communication, emerged as an essential tool for maintaining harmonious relationships. By expressing my thoughts and feelings calmly and clearly, I discovered pathways to resolution that catered to the needs of everyone involved. Moreover, it empowered me to set boundaries and advocate for myself in situations where I might feel uncomfortable or unsafe. Embracing constructive communication techniques such as open dialogue, active listening, and finding common ground, I succeeded in de-escalating conflicts and cultivating healthy relationships.

Beyond personal relationships, effective communication played a significant role in my leadership and professional growth. Leaders who communicate clearly and transparently inspire trust and motivate their teams, enhancing productivity and collaboration, thereby contributing to personal and organizational success.

Furthermore, I embraced the power of communication in networking and building professional connections. By articulating my goals, interests, and value to others effectively, I seized networking opportunities to advance my career and broaden my horizons.

In our diverse world, cultural sensitivity emerged as a vital aspect of communication. Understanding and respecting cultural differences proved instrumental in preventing misunderstandings and strengthening global relationships. Embracing cultural diversity and adapting my communication style accordingly enriched my interactions and broadened my perspectives.

The digital age has introduced new challenges in communication, as technology offers ease of access but requires a balance with face-to-face interactions to maintain authenticity and meaningful connections. Embracing the benefits of technology while cherishing the value of personal engagement, I found harmony in communication.

In conclusion, effective communication is crucial for building and maintaining strong relationships, both personal and professional. It is an ongoing journey of learning and growth. By improving communication skills, active listening, conflict resolution, and embracing empathy and cultural sensitivity, one can navigate difficult situations with confidence and assert their boundaries with ease. I hope my insights on communication can help you avoid some of the mistakes I made and build more fulfilling relationships and lives.

As you reflect on your communication skills and identify areas for improvement, consider how embracing effective communication can positively impact all areas of your life. What communication skills do you believe are most important for building strong relationships? How do you handle conflicts or disagreements in your personal or professional relationships? By learning and continuously practicing these communication skills, you can enhance your personal growth, nurture successful relationships, and achieve a more fulfilling and prosperous life.

Transition

Effective communication is the key to building strong relationships and setting realistic expectations for ourselves and others. As we have seen in the previous essay, communication skills are essential for navigating difficult situations and conflicts, and for expressing our needs and desires in a clear and assertive manner. However, as I have learned from my own experiences, communication is just one part of the equation when it comes to achieving our goals and living a fulfilling life. Next, we will explore the importance of setting realistic expectations and how it can prevent disappointments and foster a greater sense of self-confidence. Join me as we discuss what I wish I knew about setting realistic expectations by the time I turned 40. Let's dive in to discover how this valuable skill can benefit you in all areas of your life.

Setting Realistic Expectations: What I Wish I Knew by 40

As we journey through life, we face challenges that require us to set expectations for ourselves. But, all too often, we set the bar too high, leading to disappointment, frustration, and even exhaustion. Learning to set realistic expectations is essential for our mental health, happiness, and success. In this essay, I'll share what I wish I knew about setting realistic expectations by the time I turned 40.

When I opened my first business, I learned the hard way about the importance of setting realistic expectations. As a new business owner, I set unrealistic goals and quickly found myself overwhelmed with work. Despite my best efforts, I eventually burned out, and my health and well-being suffered. It took two years of slow progress and learning to pivot before I found other ways to sell my products, which eventually led to national success. But this experience taught me the importance of setting more realistic expectations and working within my limits to avoid burnout and stress.

Setting realistic expectations requires us to assess the situation and evaluate our capabilities. We need to be honest with ourselves and acknowledge our strengths and weaknesses. Setting goals that are challenging but achievable is key to avoiding disappointment and frustration. One way to set realistic expectations is to break down our goals into smaller, more manageable steps. This approach makes it easier to track progress and celebrate small victories along the way.

Another way to set realistic expectations is to seek feedback from others. Whether in our personal or professional lives, feedback can be incredibly beneficial. It helps us see things from a different perspective and identify areas that need improvement. Feedback also keeps us accountable and motivated to reach our goals.

Identifying our values is another important step in setting realistic expectations. Our values guide our expectations and help us set goals that are meaningful and fulfilling. Saying "no" to commitments that don't align with our goals or values can help us stay focused and avoid overcommitting.

Celebrating progress is also essential in setting realistic expectations. Focusing on the end result can make us forget the progress we've made. Acknowledging our achievements along the way keeps us motivated and encouraged.

It's crucial to remember that setting realistic expectations doesn't mean settling for less than what we deserve. It's about understanding our limitations and setting goals that are within our reach. By doing this, we can achieve our goals without feeling overwhelmed or discouraged, maintain a positive mindset, and boost our self-esteem.

In conclusion, setting realistic expectations is vital for our well-being and mental health. It helps us achieve our goals without feeling overwhelmed or discouraged. By being honest with ourselves, breaking down our goals, seeking feedback, identifying our values, saying "no," and celebrating progress, we can set ourselves up for success and achieve the life we've always wanted.

Take a moment to reflect on your own expectations for yourself and others. Are there any unrealistic expectations that are causing unnecessary stress? How can you adjust them in a way that is more realistic and compassionate, both to yourself and others? In what ways can you start setting challenging yet achievable goals and communicating your expectations more effectively? Remember to be patient and kind with yourself as you navigate this process.

Transition

Setting realistic expectations is undoubtedly an integral part of achieving success and maintaining our mental well-being. However, to truly thrive, we must also master the art of self-advocacy and establish healthy boundaries. In the next essay, we will delve into the significance of self-advocacy and how it empowers us to become more confident and assertive in every aspect of our lives.

Self-Advocacy: What I Wish I Knew by 40

As we journey through life, we encounter moments that demand us to set expectations for ourselves, but too often, we set the bar impossibly high, leading to frustration, disappointment, and exhaustion. Learning the art of setting realistic expectations is a crucial aspect of personal growth, contributing to our mental well-being, happiness, and success. In this essay, I'll share my reflections on what I wish I knew about setting realistic expectations by the time I turned 40.

In my early entrepreneurial venture, I faced the consequences of unrealistic expectations. As a new business owner, I set lofty goals, only to find myself overwhelmed with work and eventually experiencing exhaustion. It took two years of learning and adapting before I found a path that led to national success. This experience taught me the significance of setting attainable expectations, working within my limits, and avoiding burnout and stress.

Setting realistic expectations requires self-assessment and a genuine evaluation of our capabilities. Honesty with ourselves is key to avoiding unnecessary disappointment and frustration. Breaking down goals into smaller, achievable steps enables us to track progress and celebrate even the smallest victories.

Seeking feedback from others is invaluable, whether in personal or professional spheres. Feedback provides fresh perspectives and identifies areas for improvement, keeping us accountable and motivated to reach our objectives.

Moreover, setting boundaries is a vital component of self-advocacy. Boundaries safeguard our well-being and protect us from feeling overwhelmed. By safeguarding our time, energy, and resources, we can be more present and engaged in our lives.

Self-advocacy is not just about stating our needs and desires but also about doing so effectively. Clarity, directness, and respect in communication are essential, avoiding passive-aggressive behavior and indirectness. It's equally vital to recognize others' needs and boundaries while asserting our own.

Recognizing our values plays a role in setting realistic expectations that align with our personal fulfillment. Learning to say "no" when commitments don't align with our goals or values helps us stay focused and avoid overcommitting.

Developing self-advocacy skills may be challenging, particularly if we've spent much of our lives prioritizing others over ourselves. But with practice and support, we can cultivate this essential skill. Identifying needs and wants, saying no, communicating clearly, respecting others, and seeking guidance are steps to get started.

Remember, self-advocacy is a process that requires patience and effort. Celebrate successes, learn from challenges, and remain committed to personal growth.

In conclusion, self-advocacy empowers us to communicate our needs, wants, and boundaries effectively. It leads to increased self-esteem, improved relationships, and a sense of control over our lives. Setting realistic expectations and advocating for ourselves are interconnected elements on the journey to personal growth and fulfillment.

Now, as you grasp the essence of self-advocacy and the importance of setting boundaries and expressing your needs, consider these questions:

How has your ability (or lack thereof) to advocate for yourself affected your relationships, and what steps can you take to communicate your needs and boundaries healthily and respectfully? In what circumstances do you find it most challenging to assert yourself?

Remember, self-advocacy is an ongoing process. Embrace the journey with kindness and trust that, with practice and dedication, you can become more confident and assertive in all aspects of your life.

Yolanda Trevino

Transition

As we transition from the realm of self-advocacy, with its empowering lessons of setting boundaries and prioritizing our needs, we now venture into a topic that resonates deeply with me—cultivating resilience. My journey through life has been marked by various setbacks and challenges, and one experience, in particular, truly tested my resilience. Being in a relationship with a narcissist led to a legal problem that caused severe emotional, psychological, and financial damage. Despite the hardships, this difficult time taught me invaluable skills that helped me overcome the abuse and rebuild my life. In this essay, "Cultivating Resilience: What I Wish I Knew by 40," I'll share my reflections and practical strategies for building resilience and navigating life's adversities with strength and determination.

Cultivating Resilience: What I Wish I Knew by 40

I've faced numerous setbacks in my life, but one particular challenge truly tested my resilience – being in a relationship with a narcissist. The experience left me spiritually broken, and I had to navigate through domestic violence and unjust legal issues that were unfairly placed on my shoulders. I found myself wrongly blamed for these legal problems, becoming a scapegoat for someone else's actions. The emotional, psychological, and financial toll was significant, and it took years to recover. However, this chapter isn't about dwelling on the past; it's about the invaluable lessons I learned and the empowering journey of cultivating resilience.

Looking back, I realize that I was in a very vulnerable position, and it took a lot of strength and determination to keep fighting and rebuild my life. I learned to trust my instincts about people and situations, and to stand up for myself and use my voice. It's important to know your worth and not just accept things at face value, especially when it comes to people who may not have your best interests at heart. I found that taking classes or finding someone who has been through similar experiences can be a helpful way to learn the skills needed to cultivate greater resiliency.

Throughout my healing process, I discovered the importance of rebuilding my life from the inside out. I learned to trust my instincts, set boundaries, and prioritize my needs. This journey of self-awareness and mindfulness became the foundation for my growth and empowerment.

In the face of adversity, I found strength and determination to keep fighting and rebuild my life. I realized that resilience is not something you're born with, but a mindset that can be cultivated and developed over time. It's about seeing obstacles as opportunities and challenges as chances to grow and learn.

Self-care played a vital role in my healing journey. Nurturing my physical and emotional well-being became a priority, helping me cope with chronic pain and limitations caused by the past trauma. I also learned to seek support from positive and understanding people who uplifted and encouraged me during difficult times. A strong support system can make all the difference in navigating life's storms and emerging stronger on the other side.

Mindfulness and self-awareness became powerful tools on my path of empowerment. Embracing these practices allowed me to clear negative energy from my body, gain mental clarity, and make sound choices. By understanding myself better than anyone else, I gained the confidence to prioritize my needs and question diagnoses or treatments from doctors when necessary.

Cultivating resilience is a journey that requires patience and commitment. It involves taking risks, trying new things, and learning from mistakes. While setbacks and failures are inevitable, they do not define us. Resilience is about getting back up when we fall and finding the strength to keep moving forward.

Through this empowering journey, I discovered the value of celebrating small victories along the way. Building resilience is not a destination but an ongoing process. Each accomplishment, no matter how small, brings us closer to our goals and fuels our motivation to continue growing.

I share my story not to dwell on the past, but to inspire others who may resonate with similar experiences. If you have faced trauma or adversity, know that you are not alone. Seeking support from mental health professionals or support groups can be an essential part of the healing process. Remember that cultivating resilience is a journey unique to each individual, and it's okay to seek guidance and encouragement along the way.

In conclusion, this chapter serves as a reminder that we have the strength within us to overcome life's challenges and emerge stronger and more resilient. By nurturing our physical and emotional well-being, building a support system, and embracing a resilient mindset, we can navigate life's uncertainties with grace and determination.

Take a moment to reflect on your own resilience and consider ways to strengthen it with the following questions:

- What are some ways you have demonstrated resilience in the face of a challenge or adversity in your life? Consider the skills, strategies, or support systems you used to help you overcome the obstacle.

- What are some steps you can take to cultivate resilience and build your ability to overcome obstacles in the future? Consider the tips shared in this essay and think about how you can integrate them into your life.

Remember, building resilience is an ongoing process that requires time, effort, and commitment. Setbacks and failures are inevitable, but it's important to approach the journey with self-compassion and patience. Seeking support from mental health professionals and other resources can also be essential in developing the skills needed to overcome challenges and adversity.

If you or someone you know is experiencing domestic violence or sexual abuse, remember that help and support are available. You can contact the National Domestic Violence Hotline 24/7 at 1-800-799-SAFE (7233) for assistance.

Together, let's continue on this journey of resilience, supporting one another as we grow and thrive through life's twists and turns.

Transition

As you cultivate resilience, it becomes evident that having a strong support system is invaluable during difficult times. Building and maintaining such a system is crucial for your emotional well-being, providing you with a sense of security and comfort. Cultivating resilience has taught me the importance of surrounding oneself with positive and understanding people who uplift and encourage us. They become the pillars that support us when we face life's challenges.

In the next essay, we will delve deeper into the significance of Building A Support System. Together, we'll explore the different aspects of this essential network and how it can help us navigate through the uncertainties of life with grace and determination. Let's embark on this journey of empowerment and growth, as we discover the power of collective strength in "Building A Support System: What I Wish I Knew by 40.

Building a Support System: What I Wish I Knew by 40

When I faced a particularly challenging time in my life, I realized the immense value of having a strong support system. I was dealing with financial hardship and struggling with my mental health due to an abusive relationship. While some friends turned their backs on me, others stepped up and provided emotional support, shelter, food, and even financial assistance. My family was especially supportive, allowing me to stay with them and even helping me get my first home. Their care and love got me through some of the darkest days of my life, and I will always be grateful for their kindness.

From this experience, I learned that building and maintaining a strong support system is crucial. To do this, I prioritize staying in touch with friends and family, even when life gets busy. I make time for regular check-ins, phone calls, and visits, and I am there for others when they need me.

One of the most effective strategies I've found for building and maintaining a support system is to practice gratitude. By focusing on what I am thankful for in my life, I am better able to appreciate and nurture the relationships I have. I regularly express my gratitude to those who have supported me, whether it's through a simple "thank you" or a thoughtful gesture. I also prioritize taking care of myself, which includes eating well, getting enough rest, and staying active. This not only helps me to be emotionally and physically resilient, but it also sets a positive example for those around me.

In addition to practicing gratitude and self-care, I have also found it helpful to actively seek out opportunities to connect with others. This might mean joining a club or group that aligns with my interests, volunteering in my community, or attending social events. By putting myself out there and engaging with others, I've been able to expand my support system and build meaningful relationships with people who share my values and goals.

Ultimately, building and maintaining a support system requires effort and intentionality. It's important to invest time and energy into the relationships that matter most, and to be willing to give back and support others in return. By doing so, we can create a strong foundation of support that will help us navigate life's challenges with greater ease and resilience.

My advice to anyone who is struggling to build or maintain a support system is to be patient and persistent. It can take time to build deep and meaningful relationships, but it's worth the effort. Make time for the people you care about and be there for them when they need you. And don't be afraid to reach out for help when you need it. Remember that there are people who care about you and want to see you thrive.

As we go through life, we all face challenges that can be difficult to navigate on our own. Whether it's a health issue, a personal setback, or a major life change, having a strong support system in place can make all the difference in how we cope and move forward.

So how do we build a support system that can help us weather life's storms?

1. Identify the people in your life who are already part of your support system: Start by taking stock of the people in your life who are already there to support you. This might include family members, friends, colleagues, mentors, or even acquaintances. Take note of the people you feel most comfortable talking to and who you believe have your best interests at heart.

2. Be open to expanding your network: While your existing support system is valuable, it's always a good idea to expand your network. Look for people who share your interests and values, and try to connect with them. You can join groups or organizations that align with your passions, attend social events, or even volunteer in your community. Don't be afraid to put yourself out there and make new connections.

3. Communicate your needs: To build a strong support system, it's important to communicate your needs to the people in your life. Let them know what you're going through and what kind of support you need. It can be difficult to open up, but being honest and vulnerable can help deepen your relationships and build trust.

4. Be supportive of others: Building a support system is a two-way street. It's important to offer support to the people in your network as well. Listen to their needs and be there for them when they need it. This can help deepen your relationships and create a sense of reciprocity.

5. Embrace technology: In today's digital age, technology can be a valuable tool for building and maintaining a support system. Social media platforms, support groups, and online forums can connect you with like-minded people who can offer support and encouragement. Just be mindful of the potential downsides of social media, such as the risk of comparison and FOMO (fear of missing out).

Remember, building a support system takes time and effort, but it's worth it. Don't be afraid to lean on the people in your life when you need it, and don't hesitate to seek out new connections and relationships. By doing so, you can create a strong foundation of support that will help you weather life's challenges and celebrate its joys.

Building a strong support system takes time and effort, but it is an essential component of resilience and emotional well-being. Reflecting on your own support system can help you identify what's working well and what areas could use improvement. Here are some questions to consider:

- What kind of support do I need and how can I communicate that to the people around me?

- What are some barriers or challenges that have prevented me from building a strong support system in the past, and how can I overcome them to create a more supportive network moving forward?

Take some time to journal or think about your responses to these questions, and consider how you can apply what you've learned to strengthen your support system and improve your overall well-being.

Transition

Having a strong support system is essential for building resilience, but it's not the only tool in your arsenal. Another powerful way to cultivate inner strength and a sense of well-being is by practicing gratitude. By focusing on the good things in our lives, we can feel more connected, positive, and motivated, even in the face of challenges. In the next section, we'll delve into the power of gratitude and explore the benefits of this powerful practice and how to make it a part of your daily routine.

The Power of Gratitude: What I Wish I Knew by 40

As I reflect on my life, I've come to realize the transformative power of gratitude. There was a time when I took my health and time for granted, assuming that I would always have both. I also took for granted the people who loved me, thinking that they would always be there. However, I now understand that life is fleeting, and we should cherish every moment and relationship we have.

By cultivating gratitude, I've been able to shift my perspective and focus on the positive aspects of my life. I started by keeping a gratitude journal, where I would write down three things I'm thankful for every day. This practice helped me appreciate the small things in life and allowed me to reframe the way I approached challenges.

I've also learned that expressing gratitude to others can have a profound impact on our relationships. Taking the time to acknowledge and thank the people in my life has strengthened my connections with them and made me more mindful of the impact others have on my life.

Gratitude has helped me to find joy and fulfillment in everyday life. It has allowed me to appreciate the present moment and focus on the blessings in my life, rather than dwelling on what I lack. I now make a conscious effort to live a life of gratitude and practice mindfulness to stay present and centered.

Of all the lessons I have learned in my life, it wasn't until I was into my 40s that I truly understood the transformative power of gratitude; and I wish I had learned this lesson much earlier.

The first lesson I learned is that gratitude is a practice. It is not just a feeling that comes and goes, but rather a habit that we need to cultivate. We can do this by making a conscious effort to focus on the positive aspects of our lives and expressing gratitude for them. This can take the form of keeping a gratitude journal, where we write down the things we are grateful for each day, or simply taking a few moments each day to reflect on the good things in our lives.

One of the most powerful aspects of gratitude is its ability to shift our perspective and raise our vibration. When we focus on the positive aspects of our lives, we align ourselves with the frequency of the universe, allowing us to attract more positive experiences into our lives. This can help us to feel more optimistic and resilient, even in the face of challenges. By cultivating a grateful mindset, we can learn to appreciate the present moment and find joy in the simple things.

Gratitude can also have a profound impact on our relationships. When we express gratitude to others, we are showing them that we value and appreciate them. This can help to strengthen our connections with others and create a more positive and supportive environment. Gratitude can also help to reduce conflict and increase feelings of empathy and compassion.

Another benefit of gratitude is that it can help us manifest abundance. When we are in a state of gratitude, we are more open to receiving the abundance that the universe has to offer. This can take the form of material wealth, but it can also manifest in more intangible ways, such as love, joy, and fulfillment.

One of the most powerful ways to cultivate gratitude is through the practice of giving back. When we give to others, whether it is through volunteering, donating money, or simply offering a helping hand, we are expressing gratitude for the many blessings in our own lives. Giving back can also help to increase our sense of purpose and meaning, as we are able to make a positive impact on the world around us.

In my own life, I have experienced the power of gratitude in a very personal way. After a traumatic experience that left me feeling lost and alone, I found that practicing gratitude helped me to regain a sense of purpose and connection. By focusing on the positive aspects of my life and expressing gratitude for them, I was able to shift my perspective and find joy in the present moment. This practice also helped me to rebuild my relationships and create a more supportive environment.

Gratitude is not always easy, especially when we are going through difficult times. But even in the midst of challenges, there is always something to be grateful for. By making a conscious effort to cultivate gratitude, we can learn to appreciate the simple things in life and find joy in the present moment. We can raise our vibration, manifest abundance, and create a more positive and fulfilling life.

Here are some reflection questions that you can use to guide your thinking about gratitude:

1. What are some things in your life that you are grateful for right now?

2. How do you typically express gratitude in your daily life, if at all?

3. Can you think of a time when you experienced the transformative power of gratitude?

Transition

As you continue on your journey of self-discovery and personal growth, it's important to remember the power of gratitude in cultivating a growth mindset. Gratitude can help you shift your perspective, raise your vibration, and attract more positivity into your life, all of which can help you achieve your goals and reach your full potential. In the following essay, we'll explore ways to develop a growth mindset and embrace the power of positive thinking in order to lead a more fulfilling life

Developing a Growth Mindset: What I Wish I Knew by 40

My personal experience with a growth mindset has been profoundly transformative. Through my own struggles with various aspects of life, I discovered the power of embracing the potential for growth and improvement. I learned that setbacks are often the result of poor choices and external circumstances, but true growth comes from stepping outside of our comfort zones and taking risks, even when it feels scary or overwhelming. By sharing my story, I hope to inspire others to embrace a growth mindset and take control of their own lives, no matter what obstacles they may face.

I know from personal experience how a growth mindset can help you overcome even the most difficult challenges. There was a time in my life when I was facing setback after setback - poor choices in relationships and health, and the unfortunate dependency on prescription pills, all contributed to stress and weight gain. I felt completely alone and abandoned.

I refused to let these challenges define me or keep me down. At 40, I made the decision to take charge of my health and my life, starting by overhauling my diet and making healthy organic eating with nutrient-rich whole food, and exercise a priority. It wasn't easy at first, especially since I was carrying a lot of extra weight and felt embarrassed and awkward at the gym. Additionally, it can be discouraging to begin a new eating plan that doesn't yield immediate results. But I pushed through, recognizing that true transformation takes time and consistent effort. With patience and perseverance, I eventually lost nearly 80 pounds and transformed my health.

Along the way, I also had to overcome a dependency on prescription pills that were given to me for a misdiagnosed illness. This was a tremendously difficult challenge, but I knew that I had the inner strength to overcome it. To accomplish this, I embraced a holistic approach that encompassed exercise, healthy eating, proper supplementation for nutrition, and a mindset that focused on the positive aspects of my life. These habits and practices helped me transform my health and allowed me to overcome the challenges I faced.

Through these challenges, I learned that setbacks are often the result of poor choices and external circumstances, but that doesn't mean we can't overcome them. I gained a sense of purpose and drive that I had never had before, and felt empowered and capable even in the face of adversity. I share my story not to boast or to suggest that my experience is unique, but rather to show the power of embracing a growth mindset to overcome challenges.

Have you ever felt stuck in life? Like you're not reaching your full potential, or you can't seem to achieve your goals no matter how hard you try? You're not alone. Many of us have experienced these feelings at one time or another. But there is a way to break free from this cycle and unlock the power of a growth mindset.

A growth mindset is a belief that our abilities and intelligence can be developed and improved over time through hard work and dedication. It's the idea that we are not limited by our inherent talents or skills, but rather by our willingness to learn and grow. This mindset can be a powerful tool for personal growth and achievement.

I know firsthand the transformative power of a growth mindset. When I was in my 20s, 30s, and 40s, I faced some of the most challenging times of my life - but I refused to give up. I took charge of my health and my life by making incremental, consistent changes that added up over time. When I began to eat healthier, exercise regularly, and prioritize self-care, I transformed my entire life. I went from starting off with walking to becoming a gym enthusiast and losing nearly 80 pounds - all of the weight that piled on when I was unhappy with myself, others and my life.

Through this process, I discovered that building a growth mindset takes discipline, and it's not always easy. But by making a conscious effort to focus on my goals and take consistent action, I was able to build momentum and achieve things I never thought possible.

Here are some tips to help you cultivate a growth mindset and unlock your full potential:

Set realistic goals: Start by setting achievable goals that align with your values and aspirations. Break down your larger goals into smaller, manageable steps to make them less daunting.

Embrace failure: Failure is a natural part of the learning process. Don't be afraid to make mistakes or take risks. Learn from your failures and use them as an opportunity to grow and improve.

Cultivate self-awareness: Take time to reflect on your thoughts, feelings, and behaviors. Identify areas for improvement and seek out feedback from others to gain new perspectives and insights.

Practice resilience: When faced with challenges or setbacks, practice resilience by staying positive and persistent. Focus on finding solutions and stay committed to your goals.

Prioritize self-care: Take care of your physical, emotional, and mental well-being. Make time for exercise, healthy eating, and getting enough sleep. Invest in activities that bring you joy and help you recharge.

Building a growth mindset is a process that takes time and effort. But by making a conscious effort to embrace your potential and focus on your goals, you can achieve anything you set your mind to. So don't give up on your dreams – take action, stay committed, and keep growing.

In conclusion, a growth mindset is a powerful tool for personal growth and achievement. By focusing on our potential for growth and improvement, we can break free from limiting beliefs and achieve our goals. It's not always easy, but with discipline and dedication, anything is possible. So start taking small steps towards your goals today, and see the difference that a growth mindset can make in your life.

As I learned through my own experiences, developing a growth mindset can be the key to unlocking your full potential and achieving your goals. It's not always easy to let go of old ways of thinking, but by embracing a growth mindset, you can begin to see new possibilities and opportunities in your life. By taking small, consistent steps toward your goals, focusing on progress rather than perfection, and surrounding yourself with positive influences, you can cultivate the resilience and inner strength needed to overcome even the most difficult challenges.

As you reflect on this essay and the experiences shared, consider the following questions:

1. How have your own beliefs and attitudes held you back in the past?

2. What steps can you take to cultivate a growth mindset and embrace new possibilities in your life?

3. How can you use the power of a growth mindset to overcome the challenges you are currently facing and achieve your goals?

Remember, developing a growth mindset is a journey, not a destination. It takes time, effort, and a willingness to step outside of your comfort zone. But with perseverance, determination, and the tools and inspiration provided in this essay, you can unleash your full potential and transform your life.

Transition

While developing a growth mindset can help you overcome challenges and achieve your goals, it's important to have a clear sense of what those goals are. Sometimes, we may feel lost or uncertain about our direction in life, and that can be a source of frustration and discontent. In the next essay, we'll explore how to find your purpose and how it can bring clarity and fulfillment to your life. By sharing my experiences, I hope to inspire you to embrace a growth mindset and take control of your own life, no matter what obstacles you may face. Remember, developing a growth mindset is a journey, not a destination. It takes time, effort, and a willingness to step outside of your comfort zone. But with perseverance, determination, and the tools and inspiration provided in this essay, you can unleash your full potential and transform your life.

Finding Your Purpose: What I Wish I Knew by 40

I remember feeling lost and unsure about my purpose in life. For years, I floated through life uncertain of what that was or what it even meant, but one thing I knew for certain was that something was missing. It wasn't until a life-altering event that I realized how precious life was and how important it was to find meaning and purpose. This realization prompted me to take charge of my life and start exploring new paths that felt more aligned with my true self. Through this process, I learned some valuable lessons about finding purpose that I wish I had known earlier in life. In this essay, I want to share these insights with you and help you on your journey towards finding your own purpose.

It's common to go through life feeling lost or unsure of our purpose. We may feel like we're just going through the motions, complying with societal expectations without truly examining what is right for us. For me, it wasn't until a near-fatal event that I realized how precious life was, and how important it was to find meaning and purpose. This realization prompted me to take charge of my life and put in the work to create the changes I needed.

I've always had a strong sense of curiosity and a desire to learn and grow, but for many years I felt lost and unsure about my purpose in life. It wasn't until my mid-30s that I began to seriously contemplate what I wanted to do with my life, and it took several more years of exploration and introspection to finally find my purpose. What I learned is that finding your purpose is not a one-size-fits-all process. It requires self-reflection, openness to new experiences, and a willingness to take risks. It can be chaotic at times and unpredictable, but the rewards of discovering your purpose are well worth the effort.

In hindsight, I wish I had known earlier in life that purpose is not something that can be found overnight. It's about being open to new experiences, listening to our intuition, and following our values and passions. It can take time and patience to find our purpose, and it may require us to take risks and step outside of our comfort zones.

One thing that can be helpful in finding our purpose is to identify our values. Our values are the things that are most important to us, the things that we hold dear. They can include things like family, community, creativity, or adventure. By identifying our values, we can begin to see what truly matters to us and what we want to prioritize in our lives.

It's also important to listen to our intuition. Our intuition is a powerful tool that can guide us in the direction of our purpose. When we listen to our intuition, we are better able to tap into our deepest desires and passions. This may mean following a hunch, taking a leap of faith, or trusting our gut even when it goes against conventional wisdom.

Another lesson I learned is that finding our purpose is not a linear process. It can be a journey filled with twists and turns, setbacks and failures, and moments of self-doubt. But these moments are all part of the journey, and they can be valuable learning experiences. We can use them as opportunities to reflect on what we have learned, to adjust our course, and to keep moving forward.

To find your purpose, it's important to take the time to reflect on your values and what truly matters to you. This could include asking yourself questions like, "What brings me joy?" or "What do I want to be remembered for?" By identifying these key aspects, you can start to identify your passions and what motivates you.

It's also important to explore new experiences and take risks. Trying new things can help you to discover what you truly enjoy, and may even open up new opportunities that you never thought were possible. Don't be afraid to step out of your comfort zone and try something new.

Another helpful tip is to surround yourself with people who inspire and motivate you. Find a community of like-minded individuals who can support you on your journey, and who can offer guidance and advice. Remember that you don't have to go through this alone.

Ultimately, finding your purpose is a deeply personal and individual journey. It may take time, and it may not be a straightforward path, but the rewards of discovering your purpose and finding fulfillment in your life are immeasurable. As you go through this journey, be patient with yourself, stay open to new possibilities, and remember that each step you take is bringing you closer to a life filled with purpose and meaning.

In conclusion, finding your purpose is not a one-time event but a continuous process. It requires introspection, self-reflection, and a willingness to try new things. It is a journey filled with ups and downs, setbacks, and moments of self-doubt. But it is also a journey that is deeply rewarding and fulfilling.

Remember, finding your purpose is not a destination, but a way of life. It is about aligning your actions with your values and passions, and using your talents and skills to make a positive impact on the world around you. Whether you find your purpose through your work, your relationships, or your hobbies, the most important thing is to keep searching and stay true to yourself.

When searching for your purpose, it's important to ask yourself the right questions. Consider questions such as:

1. What do I want to be remembered for?
2. What activities or hobbies bring me the most joy and fulfillment?

3. What impact do I want to have on the world?

4. What are some challenges I've faced in the past that have prevented me from pursuing my purpose?

By reflecting on these questions, you can gain a deeper understanding of yourself and what you truly want in life. From there, you can take steps to start living your purpose more fully and overcome any obstacles that may be holding you back.

Transition

Discovering your purpose can be a fulfilling journey, but it's important to remember that the pursuit of purpose is just one part of a joyful life. Along the way, it's important to find joy in the everyday moments and make the most of each day. In the following essay, we will explore how to find joy in the journey of life and embrace the present moment.

Finding Joy in the Journey: What I Wish I Knew by 40

Upon turning 40, I came to a profound realization that I had been so focused on achieving milestones that I had forgotten to stop and appreciate the present moment, and had lost joy due to personal struggles faced over the years. However, I found joy by putting priority on myself, being mindful of the present, and creating boundaries to safeguard my peace. By working to shift my perspective, I was able to free myself from the weight of the past and focus on living in the moment. As strange as it sounds, doing something as simple as the act of cooking and preparing meals for myself each day was cultivating a sense of self-love, and I found real joy in cooking.

Some advice I would give to others who may be struggling to find joy in the journey of life would be to take the time to explore your likes and dislikes. Don't let societal pressures or norms keep you from doing things you enjoy or keep you from people that bring that to you. Don't forget to get outside and take in the beauty of your surroundings and smell the flowers once in a while. Sometimes it's the little things that bring you the biggest rewards, but we often overlook and miss them.

The journey of life is full of ups and downs, twists and turns, and unexpected detours. It's easy to get caught up in the destination and forget to enjoy the ride. But I remind you that life is a journey, not just a destination. Finding joy in the journey is something that I wish I had known when I was 40.

As I reflect on my own life, I realize that I used to be so focused on getting to the next milestone that I forgot to stop and enjoy the moment. I was always waiting for something to happen, waiting for life to start, instead of living in the present. I wish I had realized that the journey is just as important as the destination.

The truth is, life is not always going to go as planned. There will be setbacks, heartbreaks and failures, but it's important to remember that these are just part of the journey. We learn from our experiences and mistakes and grow from our failures. Instead of dwelling on the past or worrying about the future, we need to focus on enjoying the present moment.

One of the ways to find joy in the journey is to practice gratitude. Instead of focusing on what we don't have or what we haven't achieved yet, we need to focus on what we do have and what we have accomplished. Gratitude helps us to appreciate the small things in life and find joy in the present moment.

Another way to find joy in the journey is to have a sense of purpose. When we have a purpose, it gives us direction and helps us to stay focused on the journey. We are more likely to find joy in the journey when we have a sense of purpose and are working towards something meaningful.

It's also important to surround ourselves with positive people who support and encourage us on our journey. Having a supportive network of family and friends can make all the difference in finding joy in the journey.

But perhaps the most important thing in finding joy in the journey is to have a positive mindset. We need to focus on the positive aspects of our lives and look for the good in every situation. A positive mindset with gratitude helps us to see the silver lining in every cloud and find joy in even the most difficult of situations.

In conclusion, finding joy in the journey is a mindset. It's about focusing on the present moment, practicing gratitude, having a sense of purpose, surrounding ourselves with positive people, and maintaining a positive mindset. These are the things that I wish I had known by the time I was 40. I have learned that life is a journey, and finding joy in that journey is the key to a happy and fulfilling life.

As we near the end of this book, I hope that you've found the insights and stories shared here to be valuable and thought-provoking. As you reflect on the journey you've taken thus far and the experiences you've had, I encourage you to take a moment to consider what brings you the most joy and fulfillment in life.

For me, I spent years of my life focused on achieving my goals and reaching my destination, but I found that true happiness was in the journey itself. Looking back, I wish I had taken more time to enjoy the small moments and appreciate the people around me who supported me through good times and bad. It wasn't until I shifted my mindset and started focusing on the present moment that I found true joy and fulfillment in life.

So, I challenge you to do the same. Take the time to appreciate the small moments, practice gratitude, surround yourself with positive people, and cultivate a sense of purpose in your life. Remember, the journey is just as important as the destination, and finding joy in that journey is what makes life truly worth living.

As you reflect on my journey towards finding joy in the present moment, consider what brings you the most joy and fulfillment in your own life. Take a moment to consider how you can incorporate more of these things into your daily life and stay focused on what truly matters to you:

1. What are some of the activities or experiences that bring you the most joy and fulfillment?

2. How can you incorporate more of these things into your daily life and stay focused on what truly matters to you?"

Transition

As we reflect on our journey so far and continue to seek joy and purpose in life, we also come to a point where we must learn to let go of what no longer serves us. In our upcoming essay, 'Learning to Let Go: What I Wish I Knew By 40', we delve into the importance of releasing the past, living in the present, and embracing the unknown. This powerful lesson prepares us for our final essay, where we'll explore how to create healthy habits that support our growth and well-being.

Learning to Let Go: What I Wish I Knew by 40

Throughout life, we accumulate experiences, memories, and attachments that shape who we are. Some of these connections serve us well, while others weigh us down and hold us back. As I approached the milestone of turning 40, I came to a profound realization that I had been clinging tightly to emotional pain from not only past relationships but also various aspects of my life. This unwillingness to let go had caused me to build walls around myself and make poor choices, preventing me from fully embracing new opportunities and relationships. It was a wake-up call, urging me to explore the power of letting go as a transformative process necessary for personal growth and healing.

To begin the journey of letting go, I first had to identify what was holding me back and preventing me from moving forward. Alongside the emotional baggage from past relationships, I found myself entangled in the fear of being hurt again and the attachment to the history I shared with my ex-partners. Holding onto these things only caused me more pain and blocked me from new experiences and new people. I realized that letting go can be challenging and at times even feel frightening, but it opens up space for new beginnings and opportunities. It's a journey that requires self-reflection and patience, but the rewards are worth the effort.

As we navigate through life, we often encounter situations and circumstances that are beyond our control. Whether it's a failed relationship, a lost job, or an unfulfilled dream, the disappointment and pain that come with letting go can be overwhelming. However, learning to let go can be a powerful tool for personal growth and transformation. Here are some insights on how we can learn to let go, and what we wish we had known earlier in life.

Acknowledge Your Emotions:

The first step in learning to let go is to acknowledge and accept the emotions that come with it. It's okay to feel sad, angry, or disappointed when things don't go as planned. These emotions are a natural part of the human experience, and denying them can only prolong the healing process.

One of the things that helped me the most is finding healthy ways to express my emotions. Whether it was through journaling, talking to a friend, or seeking therapy, finding a way to release these emotions allowed me to process and move forward.

Recognize What You Can and Can't Control:

One of the most significant lessons I learned is that there are things in life that are beyond our control. No matter how hard we try, we can't control the actions or decisions of others, and we can't control the outcome of every situation.

However, what we can control is our response to these situations. We can choose to let go of the things that are beyond our control and focus on the things that we can control, such as our attitude, our mindset, and our actions. By doing so, I have been able to find peace and acceptance in difficult situations.

Practice Self-Compassion:

Learning to let go often involves a lot of self-compassion. It's important to be kind and gentle with ourselves during this process, and to remember that we are only human. We shouldn't beat ourselves up for making mistakes or for not being able to control everything in our lives.

Instead, we should focus on treating ourselves with kindness and compassion. This can mean taking time for self-care activities such as exercise, meditation, or simply taking a relaxing bath. By practicing self-compassion, we can help to cultivate a positive mindset and find joy in the journey.

Focus on the Present:

Another important lesson I learned is the importance of focusing on the present moment. When we dwell on the past or worry about the future, we can miss out on the beauty and joy of the present moment.

One way to focus on the present is to practice mindfulness. This involves paying attention to the sights, sounds, and sensations of the present moment, without judgment or distraction. By doing so, we can find a sense of peace and clarity, even in the midst of challenging situations.

Celebrate Small Wins:

Finally, it's important to celebrate the small wins along the way. Letting go is a process, and it's essential to acknowledge and celebrate the progress we make, no matter how small it may seem.

This can mean taking time to reflect on our accomplishments, treating ourselves to a special treat or activity, or simply taking a moment to appreciate the progress we have made.

In addition to these insights, here are some additional ideas on how to let go:

Forgive Yourself and Others:

Holding onto grudges and resentments only weighs us down and keeps us stuck in the past. Learning to forgive ourselves and others can be a powerful step in the process of letting go.

Practice Gratitude:

When we focus on what we're grateful for, we can shift our mindset to a more positive and open perspective. This can help us let go. By focusing on what we have, rather than what we have lost, we can shift our mindset and find more joy in the journey. Take time each day to reflect on what you are grateful for, whether it's a supportive friend or a beautiful sunset.

Embrace Change:

Letting go often involves embracing change, which can be scary and uncomfortable. However, change can also be a source of growth and transformation. By embracing new experiences and stepping out of your comfort zone, you can learn more about yourself and the world around you.

In conclusion, learning to let go can be a difficult but rewarding journey. By acknowledging your emotions, practicing self-compassion, focusing on the present, cultivating gratitude, and embracing change, you can find joy and peace in the journey. Remember that letting go is a process, and it won't always be easy, but it's an essential part of personal growth and transformation. As you reflect on your own journey, here are two questions to consider:

1. What are some things, people, or beliefs that you are holding onto that are no longer serving you?

2. How can you begin to let them go?

3. What fears or doubts do you have around letting go?

4. How can you address them and move forward in releasing what no longer serves you?

Transition

As we learn to let go of what no longer serves us, we make room for positive change and growth. In the upcoming essay, we'll take everything we've learned and apply it to creating healthy habits. Establishing positive routines and behaviors can be a powerful tool for personal growth and well-being. Join us in our final essay, "Creating Healthy Habits: What I Wish I Knew By 40," as we explore practical strategies to help you create the life you desire.

Creating Healthy Habits: What I Wish I Knew by 40

As we age, it becomes increasingly important to take care of our bodies and minds. One of the most effective ways to do this is by creating healthy habits. These habits can range from exercise and nutrition to mindfulness and self-care. In this essay, I will explore some of the impactful lessons I have learned about creating healthy habits and how I founded the Evolutionary Body System through my life-changing transformation.

At 40, I found myself facing a profound and life-altering moment. A traumatic event that led to a near-fatal health crisis served as a wake-up call, prompting me to reevaluate certain aspects of my life, including my habits and lifestyle. This pivotal experience became the catalyst for a transformative journey towards creating healthy habits and ultimately led to the birth of the Evolutionary Body System. It wasn't just about weight loss or superficial changes; it was a profound process of self-discovery, healing from trauma, and finding a deeper connection with myself and the world around me.

I began my path by making small changes to my diet and lifestyle, but as I progressed, I delved into mindfulness, self-compassion, and holistic practices. These acts of self-love and kindness became the foundation of the Evolutionary Body System, a program that aims to empower individuals to transform their lives through healthy habits. This journey of resilience and growth has become my life's mission, and as the founder of this program, I wholeheartedly share my experiences to inspire others to embark on their own path of wellness, joy, and self-discovery.

In the midst of my transformation, I discovered the impact of toxic relationships on my well-being. I absorbed mistreatment from various sources, leading to feelings of unworthiness. However, this realization became a turning point, as I learned to prioritize self-compassion and self-love. It was a profound lesson that I integrated into the core principles of the Evolutionary Body System.

But my journey towards creating healthy habits didn't stop at just food. I also recognized the importance of regular physical activity. Initially, I started with simple activities like taking walks and doing light exercises. As I progressed, I discovered the joy of moving my body and challenging myself to try new activities. Exercise became a regular part of my life, and I found myself looking forward to each new challenge.

As I focused on my health and wellness, I found that I was also transforming my mindset. I became increasingly mindful of my life, how I treated myself, and how I interacted with others. I learned to live in gratitude, finding joy in the simple pleasures of life. This shift in mindset and perspective became a guiding force in my life and inspired the creation of the Evolutionary Body System.

The program is not simply a weight loss plan; it's a comprehensive self-discovery journey designed to help people transform their lives through healthy habits. Drawing from my own transformative experience, I developed a holistic approach to health and wellness, addressing not only physical health but also mental and emotional well-being.

The program encourages individuals to tune into their own needs and desires and create a personalized plan that works for them. With it, you can't help but lose weight given all that you do to improve your health. It emphasizes the importance of mindfulness, self-compassion, and balance in all areas of life. The Evolutionary Body System recognizes that true transformation begins with self-love and acceptance.

Another key lesson I learned was the importance of finding balance in my life. It's easy to become overly focused on one area of our lives, such as fitness or nutrition, and neglect other important aspects like social relationships or spiritual well-being. The Evolutionary Body System recognizes the interconnectedness of all aspects of our lives and aims to support individuals in achieving balance and alignment.

The program provides resources and tools to help individuals create healthy habits and develop a strong mind-body-spirit connection. It offers meal plans, workout routines, mindfulness exercises, and personal coaching to help individuals achieve their health and wellness goals. The coaching aspect of the program is particularly valuable, as it provides individuals with the support and accountability they need to stay on track and make progress towards their goals.

In conclusion, creating healthy habits is a transformative journey that requires dedication, commitment, and patience. The Evolutionary Body System is a manifestation of my own life-changing transformation and stands as a testament to the power of self-discovery and personal growth. As the founder of this program, I share my profound experiences and lessons, including the challenges I faced and the profound transformation I underwent. My hope is to inspire others to embark on their own journey towards creating healthy habits and living a life of wellness, joy, and self-discovery.

To give you a jump start on your journey towards creating healthy habits and exploring new wellness practices, here are some easy and quick changes you can make:

1. Start your day with a glass of water to hydrate your body.
2. Take a short walk outside every day to get some fresh air and movement.

3. Practice a five-minute mindfulness meditation to center yourself.

4. Replace sugary snacks with healthier alternatives like fruits or nuts.

5. Explore the world of binaural beats for relaxation and mental clarity.

Remember, it's never too late to start creating healthy habits and living a healthier, happier life. With commitment, patience, and self-love, you can become the best version of yourself. Embrace the journey of creating healthy habits, and let it lead you to a life of wellness, joy, and self-discovery.

Reflection Questions for Personal Growth and Self-Discovery

As you've read through the essays in this book, you may have found yourself identifying with certain experiences, challenges, and lessons. Perhaps you've recognized patterns in your own life that you want to change, or you've been inspired to make positive changes in your relationships, career, or overall well-being.

Now is the time to take a step back and reflect on your own journey. It's essential to ask yourself the tough questions and be honest with your answers. What aspects of your life do you feel are out of balance? Are there any habits or patterns that are holding you back from achieving your goals or becoming the best version of yourself? Can you identify the relationships that are healthy and fulfilling, and are there any that may be toxic or draining?

Don't be afraid to dig deep and explore your innermost thoughts and feelings. This is your opportunity to take the lessons from these essays and apply them to your own life in a meaningful way. Reflection is a powerful tool in the process of self-care and personal growth.

Here are a series of reflection questions designed to help you gain greater insight into your own journey and guide you in making positive changes. The questions are grouped into seven sections that align with the themes of the essays in this book:

Section 1: Overcoming Fear and Building Resilience

1. What fears have held you back in life?

2. What steps can you take to confront and overcome your fears?

3. How can you use your experiences of overcoming fear to build resilience in other areas of your life?

Section 2: Cultivating Healthy Relationships

1. What kind of relationships do you want in your life?

2. What behaviors and habits can you change to improve the quality of your relationships?

3. What boundaries do you need to set in order to create healthier relationships?

Section 3: Navigating Life's Transitions

1. What transitions have you experienced in your life?

2. What did you learn from these transitions?

3. How can you use what you've learned to navigate future transitions with greater ease and grace?

Section 4: Finding Your Purpose

1. What brings you joy and fulfillment?

2. What do you feel most passionate about?

3. How can you align your purpose with your career and other areas of your life?

Section 5: Embracing Self-Care

1. What self-care practices are most important to you?

2. How can you make self-care a priority in your life?

3. What changes can you make to your lifestyle to support your self-care routine?

Section 6: Creating Healthy Habits

1. What healthy habits do you want to cultivate in your life?

2. What barriers have impeded your progress in forming healthy habits?

3. How can you make small, sustainable changes to create lasting healthy habits?

Section 7: The Evolutionary Body System

1. What areas of your life do you most want to improve?

2. How can the Evolutionary Body System help you achieve your wellness goals?

3. What steps can you take to start incorporating healthy habits into your daily routine?

Remember, personal growth is a lifelong journey, and these questions are just a starting point. Take your time, be patient with yourself, and trust in the process. With intention, commitment, and a growth-oriented mindset, you can create the life you envision and rightfully deserve.

7 Exercises for Cultivating Mindfulness, Self-Awareness, and Growth

The following exercises are designed to help you cultivate a more positive mindset, reduce stress and anxiety, and achieve your personal goals. These exercises can be completed at your own pace and in your own time, and can be adapted to fit your individual needs and preferences.

We recommend completing these exercises in the following order:

1. Gratitude practice: Take a few minutes each day to express gratitude for the people and things in your life. This can be done through journaling, meditation, or simply taking a moment to think about the things you are grateful for. This exercise can help you cultivate a more positive mindset and increase feelings of happiness and contentment.

2. Positive affirmations: Write down some positive affirmations that you can repeat to yourself each day. For example, "I am capable and confident" or "I am worthy of love and respect." This exercise can help you cultivate a more positive self-image and build self-confidence.

3. Mindful breathing: Set aside a few minutes each day to focus on your breath. Close your eyes and take a few deep breaths, focusing on the sensation of air entering and leaving your body. This exercise can help you cultivate a sense of calm and relaxation.

4. Meditation: Set aside a few minutes each day to meditate. Sit quietly and focus on your breath, or use a guided meditation app to help you get started. This exercise can help you cultivate a sense of calm and relaxation, reduce stress and anxiety, and improve your overall well-being.

5. Goal-setting: Set some specific, achievable goals for yourself and create a plan for achieving them. Break down your goals into smaller, manageable steps and create a timeline for completing them. This exercise can help you stay motivated and focused on achieving your goals.

6. Visualization: Take some time to visualize yourself achieving your goals and living the life you want. Use all of your senses to make the visualization as vivid as

possible. This exercise can help you stay motivated and focused on your goals.

7. Consider working with a coach: Working with a coach can provide guidance and support on your journey of personal growth and development. A coach can help you identify and overcome obstacles, develop healthy habits, and create lasting change in your life. Whether you choose to work with a coach in a group setting or one-on-one, the support and accountability a coach provides can be invaluable on your journey of growth and self-discovery.

Starting with a gratitude practice can help cultivate a positive mindset and a sense of appreciation for the good things in life. Positive affirmations can then help build a positive self-image and boost self-confidence. Mindful breathing and meditation can help reduce stress and anxiety, and promote a sense of calm and relaxation.

Goal-setting can help focus on achievable targets and create a plan for progress, while working with a coach can provide guidance and support for overcoming obstacles and creating lasting change. These exercises can be completed at your own pace and in your own time, and can be adapted to fit your individual needs and preferences.

Conclusion

Congratulations on finishing this book! In these essays, I've shared my personal experiences and reflections on various aspects of personal growth, from cultivating healthy relationships to finding your life's purpose on the lessons I've learned on my path to 40. I hope these insights have been helpful to you and have provided you with tools to navigate your own challenges.

As someone who has experienced trauma firsthand, I know just how difficult it can be to overcome. I also know how hard it is to break free from toxic relationships and start on a path of healing.

At the end of each essay, I've included reflection questions you can consider to help you move forward on your journey of self-improvement. Additionally, there's a list of reflection questions and exercises at the end of the book for you to try that can help cultivate mindfulness, self-awareness, and a growth mindset.

Remember, personal growth is a lifelong journey, and it's okay to take it one step at a time. By reflecting on your own experiences and taking intentional action, you can create a life of greater fulfillment, purpose, and joy. Life is not a destination, but a journey, and we are all in it together. So be kind to yourself, prioritize self-care, and embrace your authentic self. Cultivate healthy habits, find joy in the journey, and most importantly, never give up on your dreams.

I want to thank you for taking the time to read my book. I hope it has been a source of inspiration and encouragement for you. Always remember, it's never too late to start living the life you want, and with perseverance, hard work, and a growth mindset, you can achieve anything you set your mind to. Thank you for joining me on this journey of self-discovery and personal growth. I wish you all the best as you continue on your own path of growth and self-improvement.

Acknowledgements

I would like to express my sincere gratitude to the countless people who have supported me throughout my journey of growth and self-discovery, including my friends, colleagues, and mentors. Your encouragement and unwavering support have been instrumental in helping me pursue my dreams and achieve my goals.

I would also like to acknowledge the challenges and obstacles I faced along the way. It was through these difficulties that I learned the importance of resilience, perseverance, and the power of a positive mindset.

I also want to acknowledge my parents, who have taught me the value of hard work, determination, and resilience. Your unwavering support, even in the face of adversity, has shaped who I am today.

Finally, I want to express my gratitude to the readers of this book. Your willingness to embark on this journey of personal growth and self-discovery with me is a testament to the power of human connection and the human spirit. Thank you for being a part of this experience.

Best, Yolanda Trevino

Yolanda Trevino

Lessons Learned at 40

Yolanda Trevino

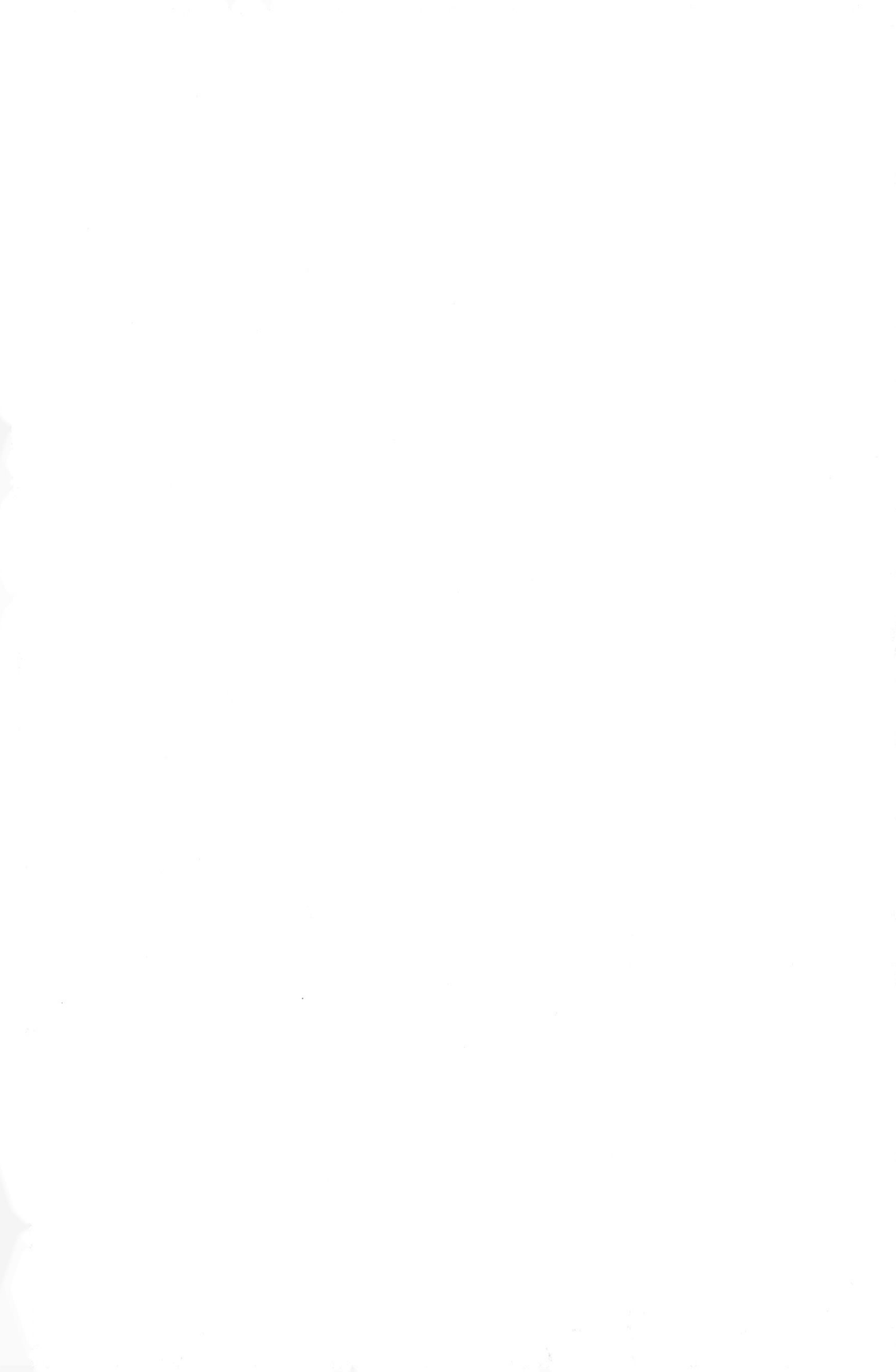

www.ingramcontent.com/pod-product-compliance
Lightning Source LLC
Chambersburg PA
CBHW071458080526
44587CB00014B/2144